HOMEOPATHIC
MEDICINE

THE COMPLETE GUIDE TO
HOMEOPATHIC REMEDIES AND
TREATMENT OF COMMON DISORDERS

Disclaimer

The information in this book is not to be used as medical advice. The information presented should be used in combination with guidance from your physician.

Effort has been made to ensure that the information in this book is accurate and complete, however, the author and the publisher do not warrant the accuracy of the information, text and graphics contained within the book due to the rapidly changing nature of science, research, known and unknown facts and internet. The Author and the publisher do not hold any responsibility for errors, omissions or contrary interpretation of the subject matter herein. This book is presented solely for motivational and informational purposes only.

TABLE OF CONTENTS

Introduction

Homeopathy was at one time one of the predominant schools of Western medicine, and became particularly well established in continental Europe, the British Empire and the United States. Its success and influence in northern and western Europe arose in part from its opposition to the drastic paradigm of bleeding and purging and surgery without anesthesia that generally prevailed in medicine from the Middle Ages on, with occasional dissent from such figures as the Swiss alchemist and pharmacologist Phillipus Theophrastus Bombastus von Hohenheim, who early in his career called himself "Paracelsus" in order to state that he was the equal of the Greco-Roman philosopher Celsus whose works Hohenheim had studied. A cantankerous and opinionated man – it is said that the word "bombast" was derived from his middle name because of his verbose and combative style of speaking and writing – Paracelsus introduced several important concepts into Renaissance science and medicine. One of them was the concept of an "unconscious" mind, thoughts and memories of which a person was not aware but which influenced his perception of and reaction to the world around him; Carl Gustav Jung maintained that it was Paracelsus rather than Sigmund Freud who first conceived of psychoanalysis. A second contribution was the concept of *dosis facit venenum* ("the dose makes the poison"), the idea that a substance could be poisonous at one dose but therapeutic at another. A third insight was that the universe and also the body were governed by an unseen life force or energy, and that healing came from infusing the body with material that had a spiritual character. At least two of these ideas have been crucial to the development of natural medicine generally, and homeopathy particularly.

Homeopathy caught on early in Great Britain because of the interest and patronage of the royal family. This led to its dissemination throughout the British Empire, in parts of which such as India it became and has remained a major component of medical practice. There and in other parts of the developing world, the relative ease of preparation, safety in clinical use and low cost of homeopathic medicines has enabled it to be used widely. In the United States, the medical profession sought to be independent of European doctrines even as the country had become independent of British rule; Thomas Jefferson, for example, suggested that the principles of the Declaration of Independence should be applied to the practice of medicine, and that doctors should look for means of assisting nature in cure and healing, and not stand in her way. The early practitioners of homeopathy were imbued by this spirit, and most of them were also disciples of the Swedish scientist, theologian and mystic Emanuel Swedenborg, who taught that the physical interventions of medical treatment had to be accompanied by some sort of spiritual or life force infusion in order to be effective. These factors made both British and American medicine potentially receptive to new doctrines concerning energy medicine.

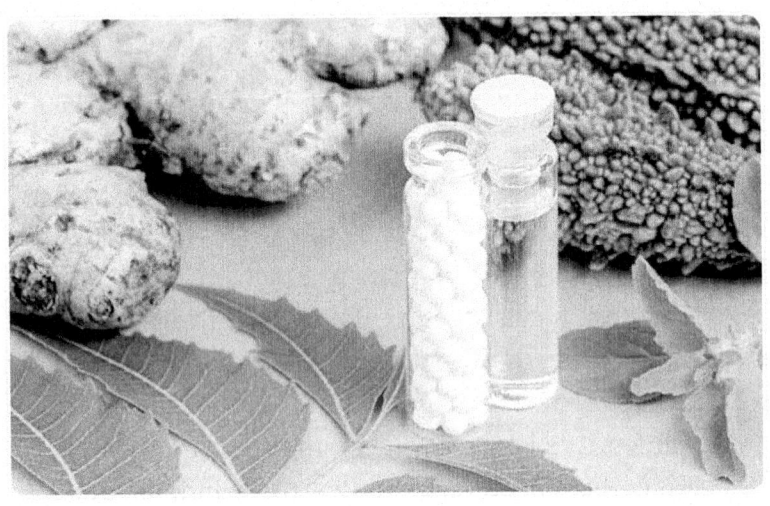

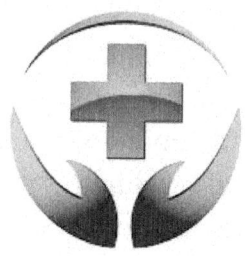

CHAPTER 1

THE RISE, FALL AND RESURGENCE OF HOMEOPATHY

Homeopathy was developed by **Dr. Samuel Hahnemann** in Germany at the end of the 18th century. Born in 1755 and the son of a skilled maker of the famous Meissen pottery, Hahnemann was sent to study medicine in Leipzig but was dissatisfied because there was little clinical experience with the sick; he transferred to Vienna but could not afford the fees, and eventually graduated with honors from the University of Erlangen in 1779. He began to practice in the coal-mining town of Mansfeld in Saxony, but was appalled by the toxic and often disastrous treatments in common use, amputation and bleeding and the administration of arsenic, mercury and other poisons. Hahnemann was an outspoken and combative in the tradition of Paracelsus, did not suffer fools gladly and as a result quarreled with colleagues and patients alike. At length, he left the profession for a time and attempted to support his wife and 11 children as a skilled chemist, and as a gifted translator of medical literature from other languages into German. His chemical skill gave him experience with pharmaceuticals of the day as well as many chemical compounds not usually used in medicine; his linguistic abilities, which included Arabic and Hebrew, allowed him to read the ancient medical texts and also to be conversant with the medical literature of most of Europe. He came to correspond with Edward Jenner in England, who had just shown that smallpox could be prevented by inoculating the patient with the similar disease of cowpox.

While translating a work by the Scottish physician William Cullen, he was struck by Cullen's assertion that the bark of the *cinchona* tree, which had recently been found to be an effective treatment for malaria, was effective because it fortified the stomach. Hahnemann had for some reason taken this, and he knew that it had not fortified *his* stomach. He decided to confirm the effects of *cinchona* bark by taking it himself, and realized after a day or two that it in fact caused all of the symptoms of malaria, which resolved after he stopped consuming the bark. Like some other physicians of the time, he had thought that most healing was actually done by the patient's own body, with modest help and sometimes hindrance from medical treatment, and he conceived that the symptoms of illness meant that the body's own healing response was not sufficiently strong, and that the response could be enhanced by inoculating the patient with an "artificial disease" to which the body could respond more effectively. *Cinchona* bark worked, he thought, by inducing artificial malaria to which the body responded curatively.

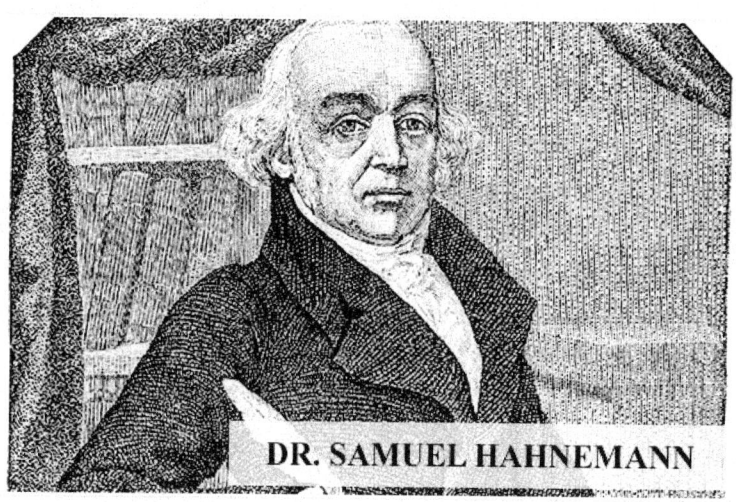

DR. SAMUEL HAHNEMANN

He proceeded to evolve an energy-based theory of health and disease similar to those of oriental medicine. In his *Organon of Medicine* he wrote that "in the healthy human state, the spirit-like life force that enlivens the material organism...keeps all parts of the organism in admirable, harmonious vital operation, as regards both feelings and functions, so that our indwelling, rational spirit can freely avail itself of this living, healthy instrument for the higher purposes of our existence". This life force or energy could be kept in balance by "treating like with like" (*Similia Similibus Curentur* or the "law of similars"), administering a treatment that produces symptoms similar to the disease being treated and therefore more efficiently stimulating the body to recover. He called this method *homeopathy*, from the Greek for "similar treatment", and labeled the traditional medical practice of giving a drug, which would antagonize or reverse a particular symptom *allopathic*, meaning "other treatment", and these names stuck. Hahnemann had to play therapeutically with the cards he was dealt, and the pharmaceutical options of his day were mostly animal, mineral or vegetable remedies, many of which he already knew to be toxic. He also had some ideas as a chemist as to what compounds might be useful, and proceeded to synthesize them. He felt too that the toxic effects could be lessened and the stimulatory effects on the life force preserved with dilution of these medicines. Hahnemann and his disciples set about administering these substances to themselves and healthy volunteers (not to sick people, he insisted, because then the symptoms of the "artificial disease" could not be distinguished from those of the real one) and recording their effects in often voluminous detail. This method was called *Prüfung*, from the German for "experiment", and these trials came to be known as "proving".

The story is told that, as he went about his rounds in a bumpy cart administering these dilute medicinal preparations, he noticed that patients seen in the afternoon did better than those seen in the morning. This story is not confirmed and patients often came to him, particularly as he became increasingly famous and eventually moved to Paris and developed a celebrity practice, but he did conclude that shaking or banging the vials of medicine as they were prepared increased their potency, a process he called "potentization" and a shaking method he labeled "sucussion". As he experimented with this, he found that the more dilute he made the preparations before potentizing them the more effective they became, and Hahnemann concluded that this process removed the toxic effects of the parent compound but strengthened its affinity for the life force.

By the time of his death in 1843, Hahnemann had developed a detailed method of clinical interview and examination, seeking to identify symptoms specific to an individual patient, which would permit a specific remedy that produced those same symptoms to be chosen for that patient. He felt that a single dose of a single properly-chosen remedy would often be sufficient to initiate the healing process, although he recognized that temporary worsening of symptoms or "aggravations" could occur, and that another dose or a follow-up remedy might sometimes be required. This came to be known as "classical" homeopathy, and its reputation was substantially enhanced in Europe by the cholera outbreaks of the 1850s, during which for example the death rate at the Homeopathic Hospital in London was half that of the allopathic institutions in the city.

Homeopathy was brought to the United States around this time, and was widely fostered by some of Hahnemann's disciples. Most notable was Constantine Hering, a German allopathic physician who first studied homeopathy in order to discredit it but who embraced it and contributed many insights, chiefly the "law of cure", that state that with successful treatment symptoms recede in the order in which they developed, and will first move from a more important organ to a less important one before resolving. Some further refinements in homeopathic practice were introduced after Hahnemann's death, in particular the observation that certain kinds of people responded to certain kinds of medicines. "Remedy" profiles were developed for homeopathic preparations, and the patient interview was used in part to identify the "type" of patient so as to select a remedy. Although in time this led to the use of several different remedies and the mixing of remedies in combination with homeopathic medications, it was consistent with Hahnemann's observation that it is just as important what kind of patient has a disease as to what kind of disease a patient has. This became known as "constitutional" homeopathy, and has led to patients with, for examples, diabetes being treated with certain remedies not so much because of the remedies' effect on diabetes as because of the remedies' effect on the patients' constitutions.

Hahnemann codified his observations and recommendations in a series of books which are still read today in the homeopathic community. The practice developed of an experienced practitioner compiling his experience with different diseases and remedies in a *Materia Medica;* some of these, like those of Richard Hughes in Britan and James Tyler Kent in the United States, are also still consulted today. A split developed in the late 19th century between some American homeopathic physicians and many British practitioners. The American school developed high potency medications through repeated dilutions and succussions. The American *Materia Medica* were often revised and expanded on the basis of current clinical experience, eventually reaching prodigious size and complexity. British homeopaths often hewed more to classical prescribing, but developed low potency preparations more like those of conventional medicine. In addition, American homeopathy acquired a more mystical bent, as some prominent American homeopaths like Kent were followers of the Swedish scientist, philosopher and theologian Emanuel Swedenborg and felt that there was a spiritual dimension to illnesses that also had to be addressed. Ironically, the American homeopaths "won" the battle with British and European practitioners but "lost" the war, at least for a time, because the decline of American homeopathy was much steeper.

Homeopathy was widely practiced in Europe, and acquired the patronage of the British royal family. There was continuing resistance in some quarters: Sir John Forbes, Queen Victoria's physician, said that the infinitesimal dosages of homeopathy were "an outrage to human reason". The American medical establishment resisted the importation of homeopathy, and the celebrated Oliver Wendell Holmes produced a book entitled *Homeopathy and Kindred Delusions.*

As in Europe, homeopathic physicians set up their own schools, hospitals and certifying bodies and the method won acceptance because its record during many 19th century epidemics and outbreaks was as good as or better than allopathic medicine. The rise of the germ theory of disease, which Kent and other homeopathic leaders unwisely opposed, and the development of more aggressive surgical technologies aimed at the cure of disease tended to supplant homeopathic medicine. The 1907 Flexner report, funded by John D. Rockefeller and the Carnegie Foundation, revolutionized American medical education and paved the way for large medical centers devoted to research and education connected to large universities. Some have also suggested that this has led to the predominant influence in American medicine of large pharmaceutical companies, and to the increasingly strict regulation of medical education and practice by large government bureaucracies. Homeopathic medical schools began to close; one of the last, at Ohio State University, was for a time next to the competing allopathic school, and was closed in 1922 when the American Medical Association threatened the university's accreditation. The medical college in Philadelphia founded by Hahnemann's students and named for him ceased offering electives in homeopathy in the 1940s, and by 1950 there were only about 75 homeopathic physicians in practice in the United States.

Homeopathy has had a resurgence in the United States since the 1970s, with as much as a tenfold increase in sales of homeopathic preparations but continues to occupy a place in British and

European medical practice. Although currently under assault in the financially-pressed National Health Service, about 25 per cent of French and German physicians continue to use homeopathic treatments. The Swiss government stopped the coverage of homeopathic services by its national health service in 2007 on the grounds that its cost-effectiveness could not be proven, but a referendum on the issue in 2009 restored funding for homeopathy by popular vote. In Latin America and particularly in India, homeopathy is widely used and is considered safe and cost-effective. Critics have ascribed the popularity of homeopathy to the influence of the New Age movement, which has embraced a number of holistic medical practices, or to the greater expenditure of time and physician attention in the homeopathic consultation than in many conventional medical encounters, as well as an implicit rejection of orthodox medical practices by the patronage of alternative medicine.

These suggestions may be true to some degree, but there has also been a resurgence of scientific interest in the ideas of Hahnemann and Hering and Kent. The Greek engineer and homeopath George Vithoulkas has proposed mechanisms for the effect of homeopathic remedies and a hierarchy for the classification of disease symptoms. He defines "health" as freedom, freedom from pain on the physical level, freedom from passion on the emotional level and freedom from self-absorption on the psychological level. The proposed parameter for measuring the health of an individual is his or her ability to be creative. The severity of disease can be graded and appropriate remedies selected by a hierarchy in which mental disturbances are more central than emotional disorders, and emotional disorders are more important than physical complaints. The focus of homeopathic evaluation is therefore the identification of specific mental symptoms primarily, secondarily the emotional effects of disease and only thirdly the physical symptoms of an illness. Homeopathic remedies are chosen that produce the mental, emotional or physical symptoms that are elicited in the evaluation, and are thought to work by imparting dynamic signals to cells and tissues that specifically change their function; the signals are thought to be encoded in water molecules that are altered in behavior at the atomic level by mixture with the remedy substances followed by dilution and potentization. These ideas accord with findings in the areas of quantum mechanics and nonlinear dynamics, and are supported by some evidence from nuclear spectroscopy techniques, and they may help to address the skepticism about how a remedy can work that has been so diluted that the original ingredient can no longer be detected in it.

Other possibly invigorating new approaches to homeopathic medicine have been presented by Jan Scholten in the Netherlands and Rajan Sankaran in India.

Scholten has suggested that the properties of mineral-based homeopathic medicines can be grouped in the same way that the properties of their component minerals have been arranged in the Periodic Table. This allows a hierarchy of patient symptoms and characteristics to be used for remedy selection, and also for the combination of features to create new remedies for particular problems. The work of Sankaran has suggested that remedies of animal, mineral or plant origin share certain family characteristics that can also be identified in the history of the patient's illness if analyzed with sufficient thoroughness, and that the most appropriate medications can be selected on the basis of the theme or "song" within the patient's detailed history. Like many homeopathic ideas, these have elicited controversy but suggest that there is still vitality in the field despite the criticisms of the medical –pharmaceutical-regulatory apparatus. This vigor is in part why the World Health Organization suggested in 2009 that homeopathy is a safe and cost-effective medical system that should be generally available.

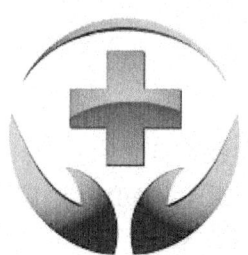

CHAPTER 2

HOW HOMEOPATHIC REMEDIES ARE MADE

Homeopathic medicines are made by dissolving animal, mineral or vegetable material, usually in alcohol, to make a "mother tincture". The tincture can be used medicinally in some cases, but it is more often diluted with alcohol or distilled water as many times as desired. Dilution can also be preceded by trituration, or grinding with a mortar and pestle or some modern replacement, which is the way medicine have traditionally been prepared. Information of some kind is transferred from the active molecules to the carrier substance through the process of potentization or dynamization. This has traditionally been done by shaking the vials in which dilution was carried out, or by striking them against the hand or a book, but is now largely done commercially with mechanical succession devices. The dilution and potentization of homeopathic remedies was standardized by the Homeopathic Pharmacopeia of the United States in the 19th Century, and the

Pharmacopeia has been regulated since 1988 by the Food and Drug Administration.

The remedies are specified as to potency by the number of potentization steps and a letter indicating the degree of dilution at each step. The decimal potencies involve 1:10 dilution and are indicated by "x", the centesimal potencies are made by diluting 1:100 and are indicated by "c" and millesimal preparations (1:1000 dilution) are labelled "M". The greatest potency is 1:50,000 dilution, which is labelled "LM" or in Europe "Q" (for quinquigesi millesimal!). Thus, a remedy with 12x potency has been diluted 1 drop of tincture to 9 drops of water or alcohol and then succussed 12 different times, and a 30c potency has on 30 successive occasions been diluted 1 drop to 99 and then succussed. European preparations are sometimes labeled "D" for decimal, and the letters and numbers are sometimes reversed, so that D5 or D10 are the same as 5x or 10x.

An alternative system of dilution is sometimes used to prepare high-potency remedies requiring repeated potentization, developed in the 19th century by Semyon Korsakov, a Russian statistician and self-trained homeopathic physician. Korsakov may have been the inventor of information technology, because in 1832, while working for the secret police, he developed a method of storing information on punch cards to facilitate automatic searching; his application for a patent was turned down and his invention was forgotten until the its accidental rediscovery in 1961. His dilution method utilized a single dilution container into which the substance was placed, diluted 1:10 or 1:100 and succussed, then emptied except for 1 part, which was again diluted 1:10 or 1:100 and succussed, and so on. Potencies prepared in this way are sometimes labeled "K" for Korsakov, to distinguish them from Hahnemann potencies labeled "H", for example, 30cH or 30cK.

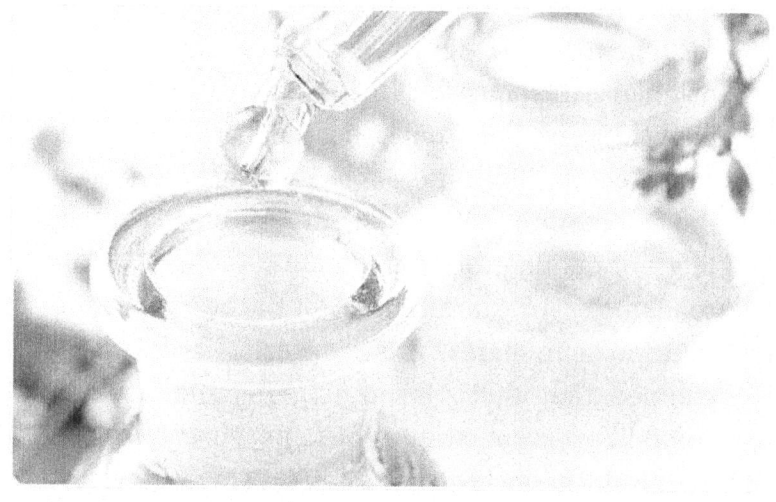

It is important in considering homeopathic medicine to distinguish between "potency" and "strength". A higher potency remedy is not stronger in the sense of delivering more medicine to its target, as with allopathic medicines. Hahnemann was not interested in giving stronger medicines; indeed, he was largely motivated to develop the homeopathic system by the excessive strength of the medicines of his day, most of which were poisons of one kind or another. Some commonly used homeopathic remedies are highly poisonous in their undiluted state, such as Aconite (wolfbane), Mercurius (mercury) or Lachesis (bushmaster snake venom), and are still toxic if taken in low potencies like 2x or 3x. At higher potencies they are not more toxic but less so, and can be safely taken at dilutions of 6x or more. In general, from potencies of 24x or 12c upward it is not possible for chemists to detect any molecules of the original substance in the remedy, and their effectiveness can only be explained if the repeated potentization or dynamization has done something to the remedy. People are often leery of taking ground-up and diluted arsenic or toadstools or tarantulas, but the repeated dilution eliminates this concern. It is often claimed that there is nothing in homeopathic remedies except water, but measurements of physical chemistry refute this, as we will see shortly. It is also said that there is no evidence that homeopathic treatments work, but studies are now being done that suggest that they do, and we will consider these below.

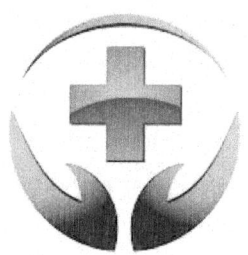

CHAPTER 3

HOW HOMEOPATHIC REMEDIES WORK

It has long been claimed by detractors of homeopathy that there is nothing in the remedies but water, that there is no evidence that they do anything and no indication that they have any effect on disease. Because most homeopathic remedies have been around for years if not centuries, are naturally-occurring substances rather than pharmaceuticals submitted to regulatory agencies for approval and have generally been used by clinicians, not all of whom are medical doctors, in office practice rather than in teaching hospitals or medical centers, there have not been the number and kind of studies done on homeopathic remedies that have been carried out with antibiotics, anticonvulsants or antidepressants. This is sometimes cited by those who pronounce homeopathy "quackery" and "pseudoscience", but this is not really fair. Experimentation of this kind is time-consuming and expensive, and neither government agencies like the National Institutes of Health nor the large pharmaceutical companies that are oriented toward prescription drugs have been inclined to fund it. Moreover, not everything that appears in a medical journal, even the most reputable ones, can be taken at face value: a 2012 study in the *Proceedings of the National Academy of Sciences* found that 2,100 papers published in medical and biological journals over about 30 years were later retracted by the journals that published them, half because of fraud and most of the rest on account of plagiarism and fraud; the numbers are small, but they attest to the increasing pressure on medical researchers to make a discovery, and perhaps to a more relaxed attitude in society toward untruthfulness. The rate of fraudulent papers increased from 10 retractions per million in 1976 to 96 per million in 2007. In addition, many reports published in good faith cannot be reproduced by other researchers and so their conclusions cannot be regarded as proven. The scientific consensus also often changes, as shown by the popular cartoon of a decade or so ago, in which the doctor gives the patient a prescription and tells him to "take these 3 times a day until you feel better or until the next study comes out." The fact is that for a long time there was little scientific evidence in support of homeopathy, but now there is some.

The "implausibility" of homeopathy is said to result from the fact that repeated dilution of the remedies make it chemically impossible that any of the starting substance is in the final dilution. This is true according to traditional physical chemistry, but materials science has shown that water molecules can form a complex 3-dimensional structure in which extremely small particles of material can be embedded. It is also possible for bubbles of gases to form inside molecules of water. In such 3-dimensional structures, information may be transferred from one surface to another without transferring any material, a process known as epitaxy. Several kinds of nuclear spectroscopy have been able to distinguish between different homeopathic remedies and between different potencies of the same remedy. In addition, very high dilutions of mineral salts similar to homeopathic preparations were cooled to very low temperatures, radiated and then rewarmed; the solutions, so dilute that there was "nothing" in them, nevertheless emitted thermoluminescence or light glow characteristic of the minerals. Advanced techniques of electron microscopy and spectroscopy have revealed extremely small nanoparticles of the starting materials in homeopathic remedies despite their extreme dilution. Highly diluted homeopathic copper, quartz and sulfur remedies have also been shown to transmit less ultraviolet light than the material in which the copper, quartz and sulfur were dissolved. These findings suggest that homeopathic remedies do in fact contain something other than water.

The other complaint about homeopathic remedies is that there is no evidence that they work. This is usually established with conventional medications by a randomized controlled trial, in which a certain number of patients with a disease are given a treatment and another patient group gets a placebo, some kind of sugar pill or inactive treatment; any difference in outcome between the 2 groups is likely to be the result of the treatment. There are many published trials of this kind with homeopathic remedies, most of them with fairly small numbers of patients. About half of them show that the patients treated with the homeopathic medicines did better than those given placebo, and the rest do not show a difference; this does not necessarily mean that the homeopathic treatment did not work, and it is not uncommon for studies of conventional medicines to show no difference from placebo. The answer in such cases is usually to study a larger number of cases or to look for a longer period of time. Many medical conditions, such as migraine and fibromyalgia, have high placebo response rates, meaning that at any given time up to half of patients will get better, at least for a while, with almost any treatment, and it is hard to "prove" that a given treatment is effective.

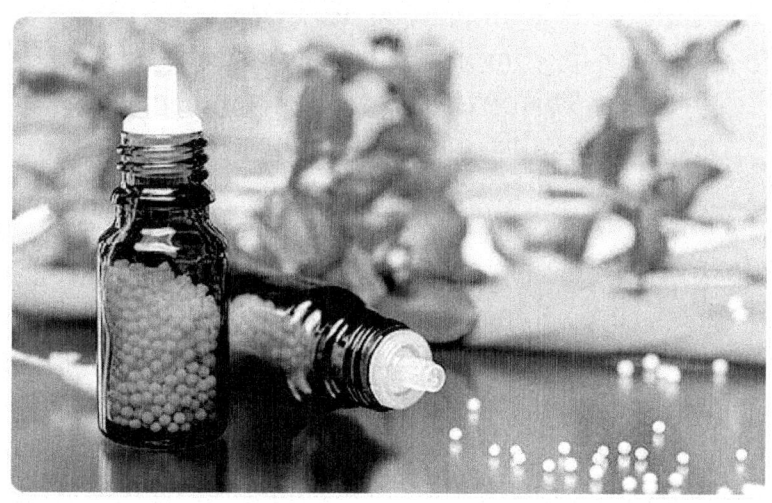

Another approach is meta-analysis, which is to combine many published studies to get a very large group of patients for statistical comparisons. Five large meta-analysis studies since 1998 have combined between 15 and 100 controlled trials of homeopathy *versus* placebo and found an advantage for homeopathic treatment over essentially no treatment. Since these analyses combined patients with several different conditions, this does not necessarily mean that homeopathic treatment will work for disease X but rather that homeopathic treatment appears to work in general. Another large meta-analysis compared 110 placebo-controlled trials of homeopathic remedies and 110 placebo-controlled trials of conventional medicines, and found that both types of treatment appeared to work better than placebo but that the statistical evidence for conventional medical treatment was stronger. This was followed by another article reanalyzing this data in a different way and reaching the opposite conclusion. The jury is thus still out regarding the relative effectiveness of homeopathy and some kinds of conventional medical treatment, but it is not the "open and shut" case that the critics of homeopathic medicine suggest. The much lower cost and likelihood of adverse effects with homeopathic remedies, and the greater empowerment and involvement in care that comes when people take responsibility for choosing and managing their own health care are not included in these comparisons, but should count for something too.

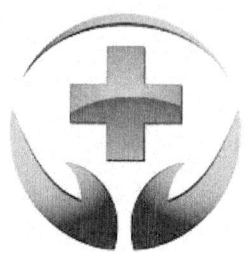

CHAPTER 4

HOMEOPATHIC CASE-TAKING

Evaluation by a homeopathic physician often takes longer than a conventional medical consultation, because so much depends upon precise characterization of the symptoms which are to be treated and the individual who is to take the remedy. Hahnemann laid out in several books a method to be followed, which is still followed today and chiefly involves listening and observing, with as few interruptions and directive or leading questions as possible. It is first necessary to identify the cause of the symptoms if known and their localization in the body; the sensations that the patient experiences, such as the characteristics of pain, must also be specified. It is important to identify what are called "modalities", the circumstances under which symptoms get better or worse. It is helpful to grade the symptoms as to intensity and frequency, and this is traditionally done by the physician with underlining one, two or three times. Concomitant symptoms at the same time as the principal ones should also be recorded.

Many physicians begin to elicit this information with a questionnaire before the consultation, and preparing an outline before the visit is also helpful, although if too detailed the physician may have to read through it later.

A well-taken case history begins with the main complaint, which instigated the visit, together with other complaints or symptoms. Additional symptoms are usually inquired for by organ system from head to foot, what is called a Review of Systems. The gynecological history in women is important even if the problem is not gynecological, because menstrual periods and pregnancy are often precipitating or aggravating and sometimes alleviating factors. The past medical and family history must be recorded as in a conventional medical evaluation.

The homeopathic consultation generally takes longer over general symptoms, which are often modalities that improve or worsen symptoms: these include diet, temperature, perspiration, influence of climate, characteristics of sleep, and relation of symptoms to season, time of day and sometimes even phase of the moon. Important dietary details are appetite, thirst, cravings for certain foods or aversion to them, and improvement or worsening when certain things are consumed or avoided. Temperature details are chiefly chills or fever, and profuse or absent perspiration may be related to these, and in many cases perspiration either improves symptoms or makes them worse. Whether symptoms are worse or better in hot or cold or dry or damp or windy conditions is an important focus in homeopathy, as is how long and how well people sleep, the positions in which they sleep and whether they toss and turn or snore and the positive or negative effect that sleep has on symptoms. Many remedies differ in their effects on symptoms according to the time of day or time of the year when the symptoms occur, and there is more information about the effects of full moon or other lunar phases on homeopathic medications than with conventional medicines.

Mental and emotional symptoms are more important for remedy selection, and first involve intellect and memory. Self-confidence *versus* fearfulness and the nature of significant fears have been linked with responsiveness to particular remedies, as have introversion or extroversion and desire for company *versus* desire for solitude. Mood is an important symptom, as is an aggressive or more passive disposition, and many symptoms are brought on or aggravated by grief and the reaction to consolation. It is important to identify through self-report or the observations of family members as many personality characteristics as possible, as different remedies may work for ambitious, compassionate, distrustful, orderly or stubborn individuals, for example. The social history may also suggest which medications may be helpful, as long homeopathic experience suggests that this in influenced by work and home life, degree and effectiveness of relaxation and recreation and sexuality and relationships.

This often complex and sometimes prolonged history-taking is followed by a physical examination as in conventional medicine. Laboratory tests are sometimes helpful, but in general homeopathic medicine focuses more on the patient's experience of symptoms and of life and the world to predict which medications will be helpful. There is no substitute in dealing with diabetes for knowing the blood sugar and insulin level, but a crucial difference between conventional medicine and homeopathy is that in the former a particular disease or symptom is usually treated with a certain medicine or a standard protocol while in homeopathy a number of remedies can be used for a given condition, depending upon the individual characteristics of a patient.

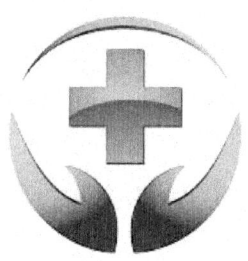

CHAPTER 5

HOW TO SELECT A HOMEOPATHIC REMEDY

The goal of the above-described evaluation is to identify the essential element of a patient's illness or symptoms, and then to match this with one of the many homeopathic remedies if possible. Sometimes a "remedy picture" is immediately established – people who have this condition with those symptoms worsened by that circumstance and improved by these things will respond to Arnica or Belladonna or Nux Vomica. More often, symptoms have to be graded, beginning with the most frequent symptoms or those of greatest intensity, often underlined 2 or 3 times in the physician's notes, or with symptoms that have been present for a long time but have now gotten worse. The causation, the event that triggered the symptom, is generally considered the most important indicator if it can be identified: asthma after being fired, depression after a romantic breakup, headache after a head injury, for example. Mental and emotional symptoms usually outweigh general and local symptoms, because they involve the whole person. General symptoms, which are particular to your body, like heavy sweating or bad dreams or painful menstrual periods, rank second because they are more characteristic of you as an individual. Local symptoms, like sore feet or cold hands, rank third because they may be associated with a particular illness but are not characteristic of you as an individual; sometimes local symptoms are individual and distinctive and then they are more important: most people with asthma do not get better if they lie on their stomachs, for example, but if you do that is a distinctive individual symptom and is important.

In his *Organon* Hahnemann wrote that "the more striking, exceptional, unusual and odd characteristic signs and symptoms of the disease case are to be especially and almost solely kept in view....the more common and indeterminate symptoms (lack of appetite, headache, lassitude, restless sleep, discomfort, etc.) are to be seen with almost every disease and medicine and thus deserve little attention unless they are more closely characterized". In a way, what is done in homeopathy is the opposite of what is done in conventional medical diagnosis.

The allopathic doctor searches the patient's symptoms for the characteristic indications of this disease or that, and when the disease is identified it is treated in a particular way in most if not all patients. Homeopathy looks for the individual symptoms in a patient with one disease or another that indicate that a specific medication will help that particular individual. These are not mutually exclusive and when both approaches are combined patient care is usually the best.

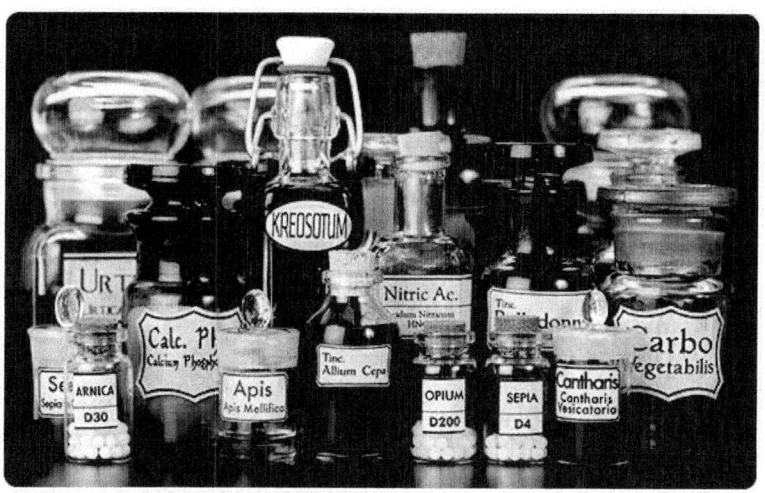

Repertories and Materia Medica

Homeopathic remedies now number in the hundreds if not thousands, and there is a vast clinical experience with them a 225-year period. It is impossible for anyone to master all of the symptoms that these many substances have produced and to recall all of the clinical uses to which they have been put. Remedies are often selected on the basis of an index of drug symptoms known as a Repertory, and the specific effects and diseases associated with a particular medicine are compiled in a reference text referred to as a Materia Medica, which was the old name for the subject that medical schools now call Pharmacology.

Hahnemann, a prodigious writer, left 14 volumes of notes on the symptoms and effects associated with the 99 remedies that he and his followers tested between 1790 and 1843. Clemens von Bönninghausen assembled them into the first Repertory in 1846 and James Tyler Kent published the most comprehensive one in English, *Repertory of the Homoeopathic Materia Medica*, in 1877. William Boericke produced 9 editions of an encyclopedic text between 1882 and his death in 1929, and several British collections of remedy experience are still consulted. These 19th century texts remain useful but are out of date regarding medical nomenclature, so new compilations have been prepared in the United States and Great Britain.

Most repertories follow the organization of Kent's huge text, which is divided into chapters on mental and emotional symptoms, all body parts from head to foot, sleep symptoms, temperature sensations, effects of perspiration, skin symptoms and general complaints that affect the whole body. Within each chapter symptoms are listed by side of the body on which the symptom appears, time of occurrence, modalities (symptoms better or worse), and direction the symptom goes in (left to right, right to left, etc.). The symptoms (pain, numbness, tingling and so on) are listed alphabetically in each section, and the remedies that have produced that symptom are listed. Remedies are generally graded within each section: if a remedy has repeatedly been shown to produce a symptom in healthy people and has cured that symptom if given to sick people, the remedy is of the second grade, while a remedy that only produced the symptom in healthy people sometimes is considered a first-grade one. Each of the significant symptoms that has been identified in a particular patient are looked up in this compendium, and the remedy that has the strongest association, such as a second-grade rating in the Repertory or 3 underlines in notes from the patient interview, with the most symptoms is the most appropriate one to give the patient. The profile of symptoms in Materia Medica collection is generally also consulted, particularly if it looks as though more than one remedy might be appropriate, to make sure that the symptoms the remedy has previously produced do not contradict the patient's report of symptoms. There are no "negative" symptoms in these drug profile: if the patient does not have one of the symptoms that a remedy has produced it may still be appropriate to use that remedy if the symptom profile otherwise matches. When the Repertory and Materia Medica match the symptoms that the patient has reported, it is likely that the "simillimum", the single most effective remedy has been found.

This method lends itself well to computer assistance, and repertory and material medica software is now widely available for homeopathic practice. Assistance in the selection of homeopathic remedies is also available through the Internet for those who wish to try homeopathic preparations on their own. Websites such as www.abchomeopathy.com, www.hpathy.com, www.webhomeopath.com, and www.homeopath-expert.com will take the interested individual through the remedy selection process. The principal manufacturers of homeopathic remedies, such as Boiron, Hyland's, Washington Homeopathic Pharmacy and Hahnemann Laboratoriesin the United States, Ainsworths in Great Britain and Boiron, which operates both in the United States and in France, have websites that can assist in selecting and purchasing homeopathic preparations. Remedy selection assistance is available at holistic health websites such as www.rodale.com. Although homeopathic remedies can be selected by anyone and purchased without prescription, it is generally recommended that the advice of a homeopathic expert be sought if these remedies are to be taken for chronic illnesses or used in combination with conventional medical treatments.

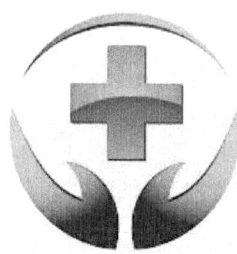

CHAPTER 6

AN INTRODUCTION TO HOMEOPATHIC REMEDIES

A recent edition of James Tyler Kent's *Repertory of the Homoeopathic Materia Medica* contains 1500 pages and weighs 3.4 pounds. It is not possible to detail the long experience with the effects, uses and remedy profiles of the many homeopathic preparations in a more modest volume, but a few pages of information on the general application of some of the common remedies is appropriate. There are 2 types of remedies, the traditional ones that are often taken one at a time and combination preparations for anxiety, insomnia, leg cramps, headache, earache, menstrual cramps and several other conditions.

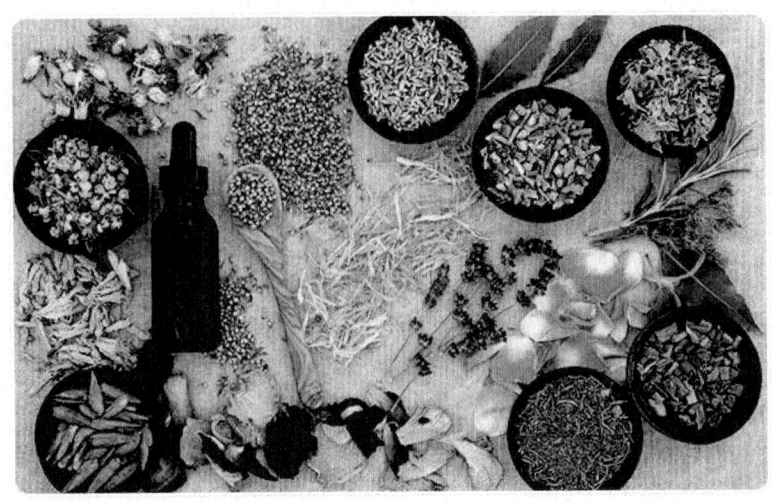

One of these, the influenza remedy Oscillococcinium, is the largest-selling over-the-counter medication in Europe. These products are proprietary preparations made by the major homeopathic manufacturers and are described in detail on the above-mentioned websites. Most of the traditional remedies are named in Latin after their animal, mineral or vegetable source, and are labeled as to potency by a Roman numeral for the degree of dilution and an Arabic numeral for the number of times the dilution was repeated. They are sometimes taken as drops or spoonfuls of the mother tincture, but are more often combined with milk sugar (lactose) to form tablets or pellets. Although the goal of classical homeopathy was a single effective dose, current recommendations are usually to take the remedies every 15 minutes for 1 or 2 hours for acute symptoms, or 1 tablet or 2 or 3 pellets twice a day for more chronic problems, stopping when the symptoms subside or changing to another remedy if the symptoms persist for a week. It is important not to take homeopathic remedies too often or for too long, or to persevere with a remedy that is not working, because this will result in an accidental proving, with medication actually causing its characteristic symptoms.

Aceticumacidum (acetic acid) is the main constituent of vinegar, and is particularly effective in thin pale individuals with waxy skin and flabby muscles. There is often marked prostration and intense thirst, copious urination and perspiration, heartburn, belching and vomiting, and there may be nosebleeds, gastrointestinal bleeding, coughing of blood or profuse menstrual bleeding. Patients are often hot and dry, with a red spot on the left cheek, drenching night sweats and inability to sleep on the back and a preference to sleep on the stomach, and may have diarrhea or croupy cough.

Aconite *(Aconitum napellus)* is used for dry cough, the early stages of fever and inflammation, initial manifestations of colds and fevers, and headaches. Patients often have a glassy-eyed appearance, are sensitive to noise and are thirsty for cold drinks, and may be in shock, anxious or fearful, frightened or panicky, physically and mentally restless or tense. Their symptoms are worse at night, especially around midnight, and in warm stuffy rooms or dry cold winds. Music or exposure to smoke will also worsen symptoms. The remedy is often used for sciatica, insomnia, irregular heartbeat, influenza, colds and fever, anxiety or angina.

Allium Cepa (onion) is used for the kind of symptoms that peeling an onion produces: teary eyes and runny nose. It is used for colds, coughs and allergic symptoms, and impatient, moody people who fear pain will respond to it. Symptoms are worse at night, in warm rooms or in cold damp weather. Sore throats, influenza, hay fever, ear infections, colds and allergies are conditions that it helps.

Antimonium Tartaricum (tartar emetic) works for cold sweats, clamminess, drowsiness, tension-type headaches that feel like a band around the head, nausea, pallor, rattling cough and vomiting. Patients prefer to be left alone and do *Antimonium Tartaricum* (tartar emetic) works for cold sweats, clamminess, drowsiness, tension-type headaches that feel like

44

a band around the head, nausea, pallor, rattling cough and vomiting. Patients prefer to be left alone and do not like to be touched; they often feel that life is unbearable, and are worse at night, when they lie down, outdoors in the damp or indoors in a warm room. Nausea and vomiting, indigestion, headache, hair loss, eczema, diarrhea, bronchitis and asthma are situations where it is used.

Apis (*Apismellifica,* honeybee venom*)* is used for symptoms similar to bee stings. Appropriate physical symptoms include burning, stinging pain, often with heat, as well as fever, eye inflammation, red and swollen joints, and sore throat. Patients are often hot and sweaty, and may have a red and glassy-eyed appearance. The remedy works for people who are angry, controlling, depressed, irritable, jealous, overly sensitive, sad, worried or workaholic, and whose symptoms get worse in the afternoon, especially around 3 p.m., with heat, in a warm bed or hot room and when touched. It is often given for sore throat, shingles, prostate enlargement, influenza, gynecological problems, food allergies, depression, colds, back pain, asthma and arthritis.

Argentum Metallicum (silver) and *Argentum nitricum* (silver nitrate) have a long history of medical use, being given for epilepsy and skin diseases in ancient times and still placed in infants' eyes at birth as an antiseptic. Painful sensations, sometimes like splinters, are a frequent keynote for its use, along with nervousness, hastiness, ulcerations of mucous membranes or discharges from them, weakness and fatigue and feelings of being dried out or prematurely old. Anxiety, claustrophobia, fears and phobias (especially of heights), hypochondria, impulsive behavior and obsessions and compulsions are often associated with relentless time pressure and always being in a hurry. Parts of the body are sometimes felt to be expanding, especially when they are painful, and there is frequently headache, usually right-sided and throbbing, and almost always vertigo; absence of vertigo with or without ringing and buzzing in the ears is felt by some to be a reason not to use this remedy. Hoarseness, sore throat, palpitations when excited or anxious that are worse when lying on the right side and stomach pain, diarrhea, belching and loud bowel sounds with craving for sweets (which are tolerated poorly) are frequent correlates. Dyspareunia (pain with intercourse) in women and impotence in men are also frequent. Left-sided symptoms predominate, and are worse with heat, at night and in early morning, with menses, after sex and when lying on the right side, while cold air, wind on the face, a cold bath or strong pressure on the forehead or scalp will improve them. These remedies often work for illnesses preceded by fear, anticipation, eating sweets, smoking or sex.

Arnica Montana (mountain daisy) is one of the most commonly used remedies, associated with pain, bruising, physical trauma, swelling and respiratory difficulty. Arnica-responsive patients often have difficulty concentrating, deny or are unaware that anything is wrong, are wary and restless, sleep poorly at night with tossing and turning and are impatient during the day but want to be left alone. Their symptoms are worse in damp weather, when they exert themselves and in particular use a painful limb, when they are touched or after lying still for a prolonged period. Arnica is widely used for pain such as arthritis, backache, fibromyalgia or headache, as well as eczema, gastritis, hemorrhoids, influenza and various injuries, burns or stings, as well as after heart attack or stroke.

Arsenicum Album (arsenic) is a notorious poison but in homeopathic doses produces burning pain, chills, dry mouth, exhaustion, fever, increased mucus production, pallor, sore throat, stomach pain and vomiting, and is accordingly helpful for such symptoms. Emotional symptoms associated with arsenic are anxiety, depression, fear, insecurity, irritability and panic. Patients for whom it is suitable are often controlling, critical of others, hypochondriacal, obsessive and may feel bruised or sore. Symptoms are increased by cold food and drinks, sometimes even by the sight or smell of food, and are worse at night or when touched. Arsenicum has been used for many conditions, including anxiety, asthma, bronchitis, chronic fatigue syndrome, colds and flu, depression, digestive disorders, dizziness, eating disorders, eczema, food and environmental allergies, headaches, heart disease and heart failure, hemorrhoids, HIV and AIDS, insomnia, psoriasis, shingles, ulcers and upper respiratory infections.

Aurum Metallicum (gold) is recommended for oversensitive people driven to despair by pain, who are particularly affected by cold, frequently congested and feel sudden rushes of blood to the head and elsewhere. They are often intensely focused and goal-directed, workaholics, serious and responsible but also idealistic and with a strong sense of duty and justice. They are often irritable and can be quarrelsome and have bad tempers, but are also introverted and taciturn and have trouble expressing feelings in other ways. They are often fearful, concerned about illness, misfortune and financial ruin, and can be hypochondriacs or deeply depressed when ill or otherwise unable to meet their goals. Patients often feel the need to pray but are not really consoled by religion, and if asked will report both longing for death and fear of dying. Suicidal thoughts and sometimes suicide attempts may occur when sick or in difficulty. Throbbing headaches at the back of the head or in the temples, frequent painful ear and mastoid infections with sensitivity to sound, intense light sensitivity and spots before the eyes and a red nose with frequent nasal discharge which may be bloody or pus-filled have been described, and daytime palpitations may be associated with nighttime chest pain beneath the sternum. Patients often have bad breath, do not like meat and much prefer bread, milk, alcohol, coffee or snacks, with either very little or very great appetite and thirst. Stomach pain, gas and constipation are common during the day, but diarrhea can occur at night, and stools are often ash-colored. Urine is cloudy and may be copious and sometimes painful, and there is frequently genital sweating with abnormal or absent menstrual periods in women and infertility in men. Intense bone pain is worse in the morning but improves with motion, and there is often knee pain and decreased mobility along with cold sweaty feet and edema. Patients often fear the night because of very bad dreams, and sleep fitfully and may awake depressed. The right side is primarily involved, and symptoms are worse in the winter or when cold, at night, when inside or during menses, and get better in the sun, outdoors, with warmth or walking, after a bath or with eating. Illnesses may respond best if they came on after grief, embarrassment, fright, lovesickness or financial loss.

Belladonna (*Atropa belladonna,* deadly nightshade*)* has been a poison, a cosmetic and sometimes an aphrodisiac for centuries, receiving the name of "beautiful woman" because its active ingredient atropine produced facial flushing and dilated pupils that were thought to be attractive. It is effective for cold hands and limbs, colds with cough and fever, dizziness, fever and facial flushing, glassy eyes, headaches (especially severe and throbbing ones), inflammation and red mucous membranes. Patients it can help are often excited, fearful, jittery and restless, and have vivid dreams alternating with insomnia. Symptoms are worse when bending down, on exposure to heat and light, with head uncovered and when lying down. Bright sunlight, motion, noise and being touched are also aggravating factors. Belladonna has been used for back pain, colds and flu, constipation, dizziness, ear infections, gout, headache (especially migraine), hypertension, insomnia, menopausal and menstrual symptoms, osteoarthritis, sinusitis and stroke. Illnesses and symptoms of sudden, violent onset and severe throbbing or pulsatile symptoms, especially with redness or fever, are particular candidates for Belladonna.

Bryonia Alba (white bryony) is useful for splitting or bursting pain in someone who does not want to move. Other symptoms include dry hacking cough and painful respirations, joint pain and swelling and great thirst. Patients likely to respond are angry and irritable, want to be left alone and do not want to move, and often feel tired, lethargic or worried. Their symptoms are worsened by bright light, warmth, drafts or dry winds, noise or excitement and any type of movement, and are often worse in the morning. A warm room may cause coughing or sneezing. It is often used for arthritis, back pain, bronchitis, carpal tunnel syndrome, colds and flu, diarrhea, dizziness, fibromyalgia, gastritis, gout, headache, heartburn, irritable bowel syndrome, sprains and strains and ulcers.

Calcarea Carbonica (calcium carbonate) has long been used for people who are pale, flabby, sweat heavily and catch illnesses easily. Other symptoms include the urge to eat indigestible things, fatigue and exhaustion, heartburn, sore throat, muscle cramps and cough. People with such symptoms are often anxious, confused, depressed, fearful, indecisive and worried, and often feel confused, insecure and homesick, needing to be in control of their situations and tending to be inflexible. Cold, dampness and drafts, diarrhea, exertion, the full moon and winter make symptoms worse. Acne, anxiety, arthritis, asthma, back pain, bronchitis, carpal tunnel syndrome, chronic fatigue, colds and flu, constipation, depression, eczema, environmental and food allergies, fibromyalgia, gout, hypertension, irritable bowel syndrome, menopause, multiple sclerosis, obesity, premenstrual syndrome, psoriasis, sinusitis and vaginitis are situations in which this remedy has been effective.

Calcarea Phosphorica (calcium phosphate) is associated with indigestion, muscle cramps, bone and joint pain and enlarged lymph nodes in the neck. Mental and emotional correlates are nervousness, restlessness, worry and the need for stimulation. Worsening factors are morning hours, cold weather, physical exertion, wearing tight clothing, receiving bad news and experiencing grief. The remedy is often used for anxiety, arthritis, back pain, carpal tunnel syndrome, insomnia and osteoporosis.

Cantharis (Cantharis vesicatoria, Spanish fly) is a famous historical aphrodisiac, and is used as a veterinary ointment. Abdominal pain and burning pain of other kinds, inflammation, blood in the stool, urinary urgency and painful urination and extreme thirst are associated physical symptoms, and anxious, irritable and sometime violent behavior are associated psychological features. Symptoms are worse in the afternoon, with movement or touch, in cold water and in relation to urination. Bladder disorders and urinary tract infections are the main clinical use, along with baldness, bronchitis and dizziness; it also enhances the effects of cancer chemotherapy.

Carbo Vegetabilis (charcoal) is used for cold sweats, exhaustion, fainting, fever, fatigue, indigestion, lethargy and weakness. Patients likely to respond to it manifest anxiety, confusion, fear of the dark, lack of interest in what is going on around them, poor memory and little or no vitality. These physical and mental symptoms are worse at night or in warm damp air, and are aggravated by eating fatty food or lying down. Illnesses for which this may be an appropriate remedy include asthma, bronchitis, chronic fatigue, environmental allergies, headache and irritable bowel syndrome.

Carbolicum Acidum (carbolic acid) was the first surgical antiseptic, introduced by Sir

Joseph Lister in 1867, and is now commonly known as phenol. Phenol compounds from various plants are also used in the herbal treatment of diabetes. Carbolic acid is associated with intense sensitivity to smell, lethargy, abdominal pain, skin abscesses, pus-filled nasal discharge, band-like headache, red face and throat, mouth ulcers, loss of appetite, painful gas combined with constipation, black stools, foul-smelling vaginal discharge, leg cramps, itchy blistering skin eruptions and arthritis.

Cephalandra Indica is made from the little or scarlet-fruited gourd, known in India as *kovai* and called *honggua* by Chinese physicians and *parval* in Indian herbal medicine. Herbal preparations of the leaves and alcohol-extracted tincture prepared from the stem lower blood sugar and may prevent hypoglycemia in diabetics, and have been shown to inhibit the enzyme glucose-6-phosphatase and to increase the production of insulin. This is usually given as the undiluted mother tincture rather than diluted and prepared as pellets or tablets.

Chamomilla (*Matricariachamomilla*, common or German chamomile) is a well-known calming herbal medicine and essential oil for aromatherapy. Homeopathic dilutions are helpful for cough, fever, heat or hot flashes, intense pain, prolonged and heavy menstrual periods and night sweats. Patients often have a low threshold for pain, and have one red and one pale cheek and sometimes one cheek is hot and the other cool. A bad temper is common, with anger, abusive conduct, bitter complaining, inner turmoil, irritability, rudeness, spitefulness and sometimes violent behavior. Becoming involved in arguments at night, feeling wind in the ears, close proximity of other people, heat and menses all make symptoms worse. Asthma, diarrhea, ear infection, insomnia, menopause and menstrual disturbances, pain and withdrawal from drugs or alcohol have been treated effectively.

Chimaphilla (*Chimaphillaumbellata,*
pipissewa, umbellate wintergreen or Prince's pine) comes from a small flowering pine tree and was used by Native Americans and then adopted by settlers. The entire tree is used to prepare the homeopathic remedy, which is used mainly for urinary tract disorders; this includes the excessive urination and urinary protein and sugar that are often the first manifestation of diabetes. Bladder inflammation, prostate enlargement or prostatitis, excessive sweating and rheumatic complaints are also helped, particularly in people who are restless, trembling on the inside and feel hot but do not perspire much. Its effects may be due to the many

antioxidants that are found in the needles or bark of most pines.

The first homeopathic remedy was *China (Chinchonasucciruba,* cinchona bark*)*, which has been the principal treatment for malaria since Hahnemann's day and which initiated the theory and practice of homeopathy by producing the symptoms of malaria in Hahnemann himself. Periodic weakness and exhaustion, coldness and shivering, hypersensitivity of the senses, throbbing headache, pale and sometimes yellow face with sunken eyes and dark circles under them, hypersensitivity and irritability, aversion to company but unhappiness when alone, nighttime grandiosity and fantasies, feeling overcome with heat and wanting to be fanned, stomach upset with gas and diarrhea, and predominantly left-sided symptoms brought on by loss or passing of large amounts of fluid (including urine) are common indications for its use. It is more often used for headaches, digestive problems and pain, but may be useful for the early manifestations of diabetes with exhaustion, thirst and excessive urination.

Chionanthus *(Chionanthusvirginica,* fringe tree*)* contains saponins, which are compounds similar to cholesterol that are found in many plants and that have been shown to reduce cholesterol levels and improve the balance between "good" and "bad" cholesterol. Its use in homeopathic trials was associated with copious dark urine sometimes containing sugar, episodic and sometimes shooting pain in the extremities, abdominal pain with liver enlargement and jaundice, colicky pain characteristic of gallbladder and bile duct disease and frontal and temporal headaches worsened by jarring or motion. It is accordingly sometimes used for disorders of the pancreas, chiefly diabetes and more recently the metabolic syndrome, as well as liver and gallbladder disease. Periodically recurrent symptoms, particularly headaches, mood changes and exhaustion that are associated with menstrual periods, are also helped.

Cocculus (*Cocculusindicus,* Indian cockle) in homeopathic proving caused back pain, limb soreness and exhaustion. Mentally, responsive patients report feelings of emptiness, exhaustion, sadness and slowed thinking. These symptoms are worse after eating, with emotional upset, in cold air, when jolted or touched, with loud noise and during menses or when sleep-deprived. Back pain, dizziness, insomnia, menstrual symptoms and motion sickness are indications for its use.

Coffea Cruda (coffee) is associated physically with increased sensitivity to pain, and with the mental or emotional symptoms of depression, despair, restlessness and racing thoughts and sleeplessness. These are worse at night or in the cold, and are aggravated by strong odors, noises or exposure to open air. Depression, headache and insomnia have been the main clinical uses.

Colocynthis (Citrulluscolocynthis, bitter apple) is derived from a poisonous gourd and can cause abdominal cramps and pain, flatulence, nausea and vomiting and painful stools. It works for people who are angry, indignant or irritable, and whose symptoms are aggravated by cold, eating and drinking (especially fruit) and dampness. It is prescribed for arthritis, bladder infection or cystitis, diarrhea, dizziness, gout, headache and irritable bowel syndrome.

Crotalus Horridus Thirst and excessive drinking, weakness and collapse, bleeding in the retina with loss of vision and susceptibility to gangrene and peripheral circulatory impairment are features of diabetes that may respond to *Crotalushorridus*, derived from Brazilian rattlesnake venom. Bleeding and hemorrhage from nose, rectum or vagina, sadness and melancholy, confusion and delirium, memory loss, dull throbbing headache that predominates posteriorly, throat pain and a sensation of constriction, coughing of blood, black or bilious vomiting, dark urine with blood, restless sleep with bad dreams and mostly right-sided symptoms that are worsened by lying on that side or by warmth and vibration may be other indicators of the potential usefulness of Crotalus.

Cuprum Metallicum (copper) may work for recurrent periodic symptoms, particularly pain and cramps, associated with tiredness, weakness after mental exertion and lack of sleep. It is helpful for serious, tense people who suppress emotions; this is often associated with panic attacks and fear, particularly of fire, and with rapidly changeable mood in adults and behavior problems such as aggression, breath-holding and temper tantrums in children. It has been used for convulsions, muscle jerks and spasms, muscle cramps, vertigo, frontal headache and stuttering, and there is frequently a copper-like taste in the mouth as well as nausea, spasmodic stomach pain in adults and colic in infants and copious, often greenish, diarrhea. Asthma with severe coughing alternates with the sensation of suffocation, and may be interspersed with nausea and vomiting; all of these symptoms are worse around 3 a.m. Being touched markedly worsens the symptoms, which are also worse with hot weather, cold air, at night and around menses; symptoms get markedly better with drinking cold water and sweating. This often works for illnesses that come on after skin eruptions like rash, eczema or sunburn are suppressed by topical treatments, and after foot perspiration.

Curara (curare) refers to a group of Central and South American plant poisons which block neuromuscular transmission by acetylcholine and produce paralysis and usually death. It came to be used as an arrow and dart poison in hunting and warfare, and was adopted and is still used by conventional medicine as a paralyzing agent for anesthesia. The extensive dilution of homeopathic remedies makes this safe for home use, however. Muscle paralysis is associated with glucose in the urine, and the production of adrenaline by the adrenal glands, which among other effects increases the release of glucose from stores so as to have a ready supply of energy in a situation of stress or danger, is reduced.

These may be the bases of its occasional usefulness in diabetes. Indecisiveness, hair loss, the feeling of fluid in the brain, ptosis or drooping of the right eyelid as may sometimes be produced by diabetic involvement of the oculomotor or third cranial nerve, shooting pains in the face and legs, menstrual irregularity or absence, weak and heavy limbs, absent reflexes and right-sided symptoms that are worse in the cold or around 2 a.m. may be other indications for its use.

Euphrasia (eyebright) was used for eye problems and as a brain stimulant in ancient times, and is associated with absent or dysfunctional menses, inflammation after injury and mucus production. It has no particular mental or emotional correlates, but symptoms are worse indoors, with bright lights, in warmth and during evening hours. It is used for eye problems and headaches as of old, but also for allergies and hay fever, colds, constipation and prostate disorders.

Ferrum Phosphoricum (iron phosphate) is effective for abdominal pain, exhaustion, lack of appetite, pallor, paralysis and vomiting, especially in nervous and sensitive people. Potentially responsive symptoms are worse at night, after eating and between 4 and 6 a.m. Rapid movement, jarring, being touched, and being in the sun or heat will also worsen them. Anemia, arthritis, back pain, bronchitis, colds and flu, diarrhea, dizziness, earache and ear infection, fibromyalgia, hay fever, miscarriages and stroke have been treated with this.

Gelsemium *(Gelsemium sempervivens, jasmine)* is associated with chills, exhaustion, fatigue, fever, pulsating headaches (especially at the back of the head) and sleepiness with heavy and drooping eyelids. Patients are often anxious but apathetic about their illness, depressed, dull, fearful, nervousness and have racing thoughts or phobias, decreased or blurred vision (especially during headaches), tremor and weakness. They often feel inadequate and are afraid to be alone Mental exertion, excitement or bad news worsen symptoms, as do dampness, fog, hot sun or open air. Coffee, alcohol or stimulant drugs are also aggravating. It has been used for allergies, anxiety, arthritis, chronic fatigue, depression, diarrhea, dizziness, fibromyalgia, influenza, migraine and tension headache and stroke. It is also strengthening during cancer chemotherapy or childbirth.

Helleborus Niger *(*black hellbore or Christmas rose*)* was used by the Greeks and Romans to treat mental problems, and Socrates and other philosophers drank an infusion of it to maintain their stamina and concentration during prolonged debates. It is actually a buttercup rather than a rose, and is no longer used much in herbal medicine because of concerns about its toxicity; after repeated homeopathic dilutions it is safe and used to treat grief, depression and lethargy, especially in the evening between 4 and 8 p.m., as well as difficulty thinking, concentrating and remembering. This has been used for the cognitive and memory problems, probably related to disease of small blood vessels and reduction of brain circulation that is an increasingly recognized problem in long-term diabetes.

Hepar Sulphuris *(Calcarea Suphuratum Hahnemanii,* calcium sulfate*)* is one of several homeopathic medicines developed by Hahnemann himself, in this case from combining oyster shell calcium and flowers of sulphur, which was brimstone in the Bible. Associated physical symptoms include chills, dry cough, fever, joint pain, mucus production which cannot be expectorated, sore throat, swollen lymph nodes and foul-smelling discharges. Patients are very sensitive and easily offended, irritable, impulsive and anxious, and are made worse by cold air, cold food or drinks, noise or touch, and by being bothered or uncovered. Traditional uses include acne, allergies, allergies, anxiety, bronchitis, colds, diarrhea, ear infections and earache, eczema, sinusitis and ulcers.

Hypericum *(Hypericum Perforatum,* St. John's wort*)* is an old herbal medicine for pain and injury, and is useful homeopathically for indigestion, nausea, nerve pain (especially lightning-like or shooting) and puncture wounds. Patients are often depressed and inattentive, forgetful, sleepy or seemingly in shock. Symptoms are worsened by cold and damp, fog, warm stuffy rooms or when touched or uncovered. It is useful for back pain, depression, diarrhea, headache, hemorrhoids, impotence and injuries (sprains, strains, punctures, contusions and injury to nerves or spine).

Ignatia Amara *(*St. Ignatius bean*)* is associated with drowsiness, dry cough, fever and chills, stabbing headache, sore throat and frequent yawning. Patients cry easily, have prolonged or unresolved grief and are often angry or resentful and have had some past emotional trauma. Sighing, sentimentality, weepiness, and the sensation of a lump in the throat are often present. Consolation is poorly received despite evident emotional distress, and strong emotions as well as strong smells make symptoms worse. Other aggravating factors are cold air, rain, winter, morning hours, exposure to smoke or use of alcohol, coffee or tobacco. It has been used for anxiety, asthma, back pain, chronic fatigue, colds and flu, constipation, depression, eating disorders, hemorrhoids, insomnia, migraine and other chronic headaches, menstrual problems as well as menopause and obesity.

Ipecacuanha (ipecacuanha root) is a highly nauseating Brazilian root used in conventional medicine to induce vomiting after poisoning (Ipecac). It is used homeopathically for bleeding, expectorated blood, cough, fever, indigestion, nausea and vomiting, red face, swelling and weakness. Associated mental and emotional symptoms are anxiety, argumentativeness, irritability, and moroseness; patients are often contemptuous of others but fearful of death. Symptoms are worse in the winter and when lying down, moving or hot. It is used for asthma, back pain, bleeding, adverse effects of chemotherapy, migraine, morning sickness in pregnancy and motion sickness.

Kali Bichromium (potassium bichromate) was another invention of Dr. Hahnemann, and is used for productive coughs, joint pain, postnasal drip, nasal and other discharges that are thick and stringy and hypersensitivity to pain. Patients whom it helps are often anxious and irritable, and symptoms are worse in the morning and in cold weather, as well as with loud noise or touching. It is prescribed for arthritis, bronchitis,

colds with congestion, earaches and ear infections, migraine and other headaches (especially if confined to one area), sinusitis and vaginitis.

Kali Carbonicum (potassium carbonate) is associated physically with dizziness, headaches (especially before menstrual periods), nasal congestion, muscle stiffness, and phlegm, and mentally with fear of the future, feeling overwhelmed, irritability, nervousness and unhappiness. Coffee, cold weather, hot drinks, being touched and changes in weather make symptoms worse. Dizziness, headache, premenstrual tension and upper respiratory infections and bronchitis are common uses.

Lac Defloratum (skim milk) was first used medically in the nutritional treatment of diabetes and kidney disease in the 19th century. It is effective for various illnesses characterized by profuse urination, often with thick milky urine containing protein. Headache, usually throbbing and with nausea, vomiting and visual symptoms and constipation are other associated symptoms that may suggest its use.

Lachesis (Lachesis Mutus, bushmaster snake venom) is a snake poison also used on arrows by

South American tribes, and in homeopathic doses caused fatigue, fever, hot flashes, palpitations, sore throat and weak heart. It is particularly effective for left-sided symptoms, and in people who are depressed, excitable, irritable, jealous, sensitive, suspicious or talkative by nature. Symptoms are worse after alcohol use, bright light, heat, touch and awakening in the morning, and tight clothing or anything around the neck is particularly intolerable. It is used for asthma, chronic fatigue, headache, heavy periods, hemorrhoids, hypertension, kidney stones, menopause, migraine and premenstrual tension, especially when symptoms begin on the left side or are worse there.

Lacticum Acidum (lactic acid) was frequently used for diabetes in the 19th century, along with morning sickness, breast pain and rheumatism. Associated symptoms are sore throat, breast pain, nausea, morning sickness, joint pain and copious urination. There is often dyshydrosis (severe foot sweating) and dysbiosis (intestinal overgrowth by harmful bacteria) with resultant stomach and bowel symptoms. The tongue is often white and coated, and there is a coppery taste in the mouth along with hoarseness. Patients are often pale, cold and melancholy, feel weak and are averse to mental or physical activity, feeling sore and exhausted as if after intense exertion even though they have not.

Ledum (*Ledum Palustre,* marsh tea*)* is effective for abscesses, bleeding and bruising, chills and coldness headaches, joint pain, puncture wounds, strains, stings and bites and for throbbing pain generally. Patients often experience anger, anxiety, glumness, impatience and timidity, and often want to be left alone. Heat, lying down, moving about, being in a warm room or covered up and nighttime will worsen symptoms. Alcohol abuse, arthritis, bronchitis, colds and flu, gout, headaches, infections (especially bladder or kidney), puncture wounds and sprains and strains have responded to this.

Lycopodium (*Lycopodium Clavatum,* club moss*)* was traditionally called "wolf's claw" because of its appearance, and is associated with the formation of thick mucus, coughs and fevers, headache, indigestion, prostate enlargement and prostatitis, puncture wounds and skin eruptions, as well as anxiety, fear of failure, hypochondriasis, impatience, feelings of inferiority or superiority, insecurity, lack of self-control, mental exhaustion, nervousness and secretiveness. Symptoms are worse when cold or when covered up as well as at night, when wearing tight clothing and in stuffy rooms, and are also aggravated by coughing, eating irregularly or eating too much. Many illnesses have been treated with *lycopodium*, including anxiety, asthma, baldness, bronchitis, chronic fatigue, colds and flu, constipation, diabetes, various digestive disorders (colitis, Crohn's disease, food allergies, heartburn, irritable bowel syndrome), impotence, insomnia, macular degeneration, migraine, premenstrual stress, sinusitis, multiple skin disorders (eczema, psoriasis, rosacea, seborrhea) and urinary tract disorders (bladder and kidney infections, cystitis, kidney stones, prostatic enlargement).

Magnesia Phosphoric (magnesium phosphate) in homeopathic proving caused aches and pains, muscle cramps and spasms and nausea, and patients also reported difficulty thinking clearly and tiredness, and complained, moaned and groaned. Symptoms were worse at night or in the cold, and were aggravated by drafts or being touched. Back pain, dizziness, earaches and ear infections, headaches, leg cramps, menstrual pain and morning sickness have been successfully treated.

Mercurius (*MercuriuSolubilis,* mercury or quicksilver) is ordinarily highly toxic, but in homeopathic doses works for dry and sore

throats, inflamed eyes, fever, neuralgia, and thirst. Patients are often anxious, dull, irritable, nervous, timid or suspicious, and lack will power or have poor concentration and memory. Night, warmth of the bed, dampness, daylight and changes in temperature make symptoms worse. It is used for back pain, colds, colitis, ear infections, fibromyalgia, sinus infections, ulcers and vaginitis.

Moschus (*Moschus Moschiferus,* deer musk*)* is produced by an abdominal gland of the musk deer and is used as a scent and fixative in the perfume industry. It is very intense, and can cause faintness and dizziness or even loss of consciousness in susceptible individuals. Hahnemann felt that people who used scents and perfumes put themselves at risk for chronic diseases by suppressing the immune system, and developed a homeopathic preparation of the scent for immune stimulation and to revive the faint and fainting. It has been suggested for use in recurrent hypoglycemia or symptoms of low blood sugar that are not necessarily accompanied by blood sugar decrease, and may by regulating the immune system lessen the likelihood of developing type 1 diabetes, in which antibodies to insulin-producing beta cells in the pancreas have been found. Copious amounts of dilute urine, often accompanied by thirst, are potential indications for its use. Asthma with mucus production, anxiety, productive cough, flatulence, hysteria and mood swings are other potential indicators for it.

Natrum Muriaticum (sodium chloride) is associated with cravings, fever, headache, menstrual irregularity, nausea and vomiting, clear nasal discharge, sore throat, thirst, weakness and a whooping cough. Associated mental and emotional symptoms include brooding sadness, difficulty expressing feelings, depressions, feelings of abandonment, grief, impatience, loneliness, low spirits and moodiness, a sense of doom, sentimentality and tearfulness and sobbing. These are worsened by crying in front of others or being consoled by them, as well as extreme cold, being in the sun or in drafts, morning hours, hearing music, being in a warm room or being jarred or jostled. Anemia, anxiety, asthma, back pain, chronic fatigue, cold and flu, constipation, diarrhea, dizziness, eczema and allergies, hemorrhoids, hypertension, irritable bowel syndrome, menopause, menstrual symptoms, migraine, motion sickness, obesity, psoriasis, sciatica, ulcers and vaginitis have been successfully treated.

Niticum Acidum (nitric acid) is frequently prescribed for the keynote symptoms of

71

weakness, trembling and sharp pain that comes and goes suddenly. It is also helpful for chills in a warm room or environment, fear of the cold, copious and strong-smelling urine, profuse sweating especially at night and bleeding from nose, rectum and vagina. Patients are often fearful of disease, doubt they will ever recover and consult many physicians; they are also often angry, irritable, resentful and malicious, tending to blame others but worried and sometimes hopeless. As diseases progress, they experience presentiments of death and loss of memory, and report severe sleep problems. Nighttime awakening often occurs around 2 a.m., and there are alternately band-like and throbbing headaches, sometimes with vertigo. Lymph nodes are often swollen, and nasal discharge is frequent, often infected and bad smelling. There is coughing during the night and stitching pain interfering with breathing during the day, along with heart palpitations and anxiety about these. People helped by nitric acid often crave fat and salt, are averse to meat, bread and milk, and sometimes have the urge to eat indigestible things like dirt or chalk. Stabbing abdominal pain and nausea often follows eating, and stools are hard, very smelly and painful, with pain after defecation and often hemorrhoids. Urine is dark and feels cold, and is sometimes bloody, and urethral irritation and discharge in men and vaginal itching in women may occur after sex, along with genital warts. Joints and limbs are painful, and patients often feel as if walking on needles, often with very sweaty feet. Symptoms are worse in the evening and at night, especially after 2 a.m., and are aggravated by cold, touch and being awakened, while warmth and passive motion such as riding in a car improve them; symptoms are predominantly left-sided, and will often disappear after a discharge from mucous membranes, like runny or bloody nose or vaginal discharge of bleeding.

Nux Vomica *(Strychnos Nux vomica,* poison nut) contains strychnine and is poisonous in pure form, but is safe when highly diluted as a homeopathic remedy. It works on chills and fevers, coughs, flatulence, heartburn and other indigestion, labor pain, nausea and vomiting and phlegm. Patients often manifest aggressive behavior and are angry, anxious, indignant, irritable, spiteful or stubborn; they ate often highly competitive, intimidating to others, self-centered and jealous, but are fearful or sensitive to criticism and often feel stressed out. They dislike being touched and sometimes eat and drink (especially alcohol) to excess, and symptoms are worse with hangovers or overeating, particularly of hot spicy food. They are also intolerant of noise and bright lights, and are worse when touched or awakened, or in cold winds or warm rooms. Alcoholism and drug addiction, asthma, back pain, bladder infections and cystitis, constipation, chronic fatigue, colds and flu, diarrhea, digestive disorders (colitis, Crohn's disease, irritable bowel syndrome) dizziness, endometriosis, environmental allergies, fibroids of the uterus, gout, hay fever, headaches, heart disease, hemorrhoids, hypertension, insomnia, kidney stones, menopause and menstrual pain and tension, morning sickness, motion sickness, multiple sclerosis and the physical effects of stress have been effectively treated.

Phosphoricum Acidum (phosphoric acid) is widely used in soft drinks, and in homeopathic trials caused exhaustion and weakness with profuse sweating and flushing, pallor, emaciation and coldness. Patients are indifferent and apathetic, forgetful, dizzy and often lethargic and sometimes in a stupor. Hair loss and headache are associated with dry eyes and nose, a bitter taste in the mouth, lack of appetite but craving for drinks, distended abdomen with gas and painless diarrhea that is worse in the summer. Urine is copious in amount and milky in appearance, and impotence and loss of interest in sex are frequent. Limb weakness, burning or shooting pain and incoordination are present, sometimes formication (the sensation of ants crawling over the skin). Symptoms predominate on the right side and are worse at night, in cold and drafts, with mental exertion, and with light or noise but better after sleep, in heat or with motion. Symptoms also often begin after grief, worry, shock, mental exertion or bad news and may follow fluid loss or illness.

Phosphorus is used for burning pain, chills, cough with and without phlegm, deafness, fever, headache, indigestion, joint and muscle pain, laryngitis, sore throat, swelling around the eyes, excessive thirst (especially for ice cold drinks) and vomiting. It is also associated with anxiety, a tendency to bottle up or hold in emotions, fear of being alone, worry about becoming insane, indifference to illness, nervous attention, efforts to obtain approval and love and suicidal ideas or behavior. Symptoms are worsened by cold drafts, mental effort, noises, odors, warm food and drinks and changes in weather, and are particularly worse in the evening. Many conditions have been improved by *phosphorus*: Alzheimer's disease, anemia, anxiety, arthritis, asthma, bleeding disorders and hemorrhage, bronchitis, cataracts, chronic fatigue, colds and flu, constipation, depression, diabetes, dizziness, eczema, fibromyalgia, food and environmental allergies, gastritis, glaucoma, hay fever, hearing loss, heart disease and heart failure, hemorrhoids, hypertension, insomnia, irritable bowel syndrome, migraine, morning sickness, obesity, psoriasis, respiratory infections, rheumatoid arthritis, and ulcers.

Picrinicum Acidum (picric acid) is another phenol compound, and may help diabetes by enhancing the effects of insulin. It is associated with general burnout, with mental, emotional and physical weakness, exhaustion and burning pain. Sleepiness and difficulty concentrating during the day are accompanied by sleeplessness at night, and there is often severe headache when stressed or with sorrow. Patients, especially men, often feel sexual excitement and strong desire, may masturbate frequently and have spontaneous erections and sometimes priapism or prolonged painful erection. There is back pain and burning pain in the legs, sometimes associated with weakness and occasionally progressing to paralysis, and also with writer's cramp. Exertion, stress, grief, heat and stools make symptoms worse, and open air, cool weather, lying down and firm pressure on the head during headache make them better. This remedy works particularly for illnesses that come on after overexertion.

Podophyllum *(Podophyllum Peltatum,* may apple*)* is associated with abdominal main, mucus in bowel movements, stomach cramps and growling, faintness, joint and muscle stiffness, sudden urgency to defecate, thirst for cold drinks and weakness. Depression, excitability, sleeps vocalization and headaches.

Plumbum Metallicum (lead) is a homeopathic dilution of a serious poison, and is associated with progressive slowness, weakness, wasting away and anemia. Mental dullness, apathy, anxiety, sadness, suspicion and fear of being poisoned are frequent symptoms, and *plumbum* candidates are often people who have been self-centered and enjoyed luxury in the past but are now unable to do so on account of health or finances, or who have previously enjoyed risk-taking behavior. The facial skin is often oily and the cheeks sunken, and parotid and salivary glands are swollen and inflamed. There are blue lines under the teeth on the gums, colicky abdominal pain radiating to other areas is common and patients strongly desire fried or salty food. The abdomen is retracted, and people feel that it is being drawn back toward the spine and have constipation and sometimes spasms of the anus. There is often much urination, but urine can be retained due to bladder paralysis and kidneys may be chronically irritated. Women are prone to miscarriage, hypersensitivity of the vagina, vaginismus (vaginal spasm after sex) and swollen painful breasts, while men may have impotence. Lightning-like pain is present in the extremities, which may be weak and after time atrophied; in particular, foot drop and wrist drop are present; pain is worse at night and the limbs are often sensitive when touched. Exertion, motion, cold air, evening and night, being touched and fasting aggravate symptoms; hard pressure on painful limbs, rubbing painful areas, stretching limbs or heat improve them.

Pulsatilla (*Pulsatilla Pratensis,* wind flower) is derived from an ancient medicinal plant that blossoms around Easter and is therefore sometimes called pasque flower. Its homeopathic use resulted in burning vaginal discharge, eye inflammation, hacking cough, heartburn, nausea, pain that moves from joint to joint, eye swelling, yellow or greenish discharges, menstrual disturbance and lack of thirst. Associated mental or emotional symptoms include depression, fear, moodiness, sensitivity and tearfulness; patients are often weepy and clingy, avoid concentration, long for attention and are slow, gentle and quiet in disposition. Symptoms are worse in the evening, when lying down at night, or when moving rapidly, and are aggravated by sunlight, heat, changes in temperature, warm rooms or beds and eating rich or fatty foods. Historically used much more for women than for men, and often given to children, it has been effective for acne, allergies, arthritis, asthma, back pain (especially sciatica), bronchitis, cataracts, chronic fatigue, colds and flu, cystitis, depression (especially post-partum), diarrhea, digestive disorders, dizziness, earaches and ear infections, fibromyalgia, hay fever, headache, hemorrhoids, labor pain, menopause and menstrual tension, morning sickness, prostate enlargement in men, sinusitis and vaginitis.

Rhus Toxicodendron (poison ivy) works for acute pain and arthritis pain with initial attempts to move, cold sores, fever, itching, joint and muscle pain generally, rash, sore throat and sprains and strains. Patients are restless and are often depressed and cry easily, and may be irritable, lonely or nervous. They are often very thirsty, especially for cold drinks. Cold drinks, damp and cold weather, drafts and wet conditions aggravate symptoms, and they are often worse in bed at night. Poison ivy is classically treated with this, along with back pain, carpal tunnel syndrome, colds and flu, depression, dizziness, gout, headaches, shingles, sprains and strains and temporomandibular joint dysfunction, as well as various skin conditions (acne, hives, psoriasis, rosacea).

Ruta *(Ruta Graveolens,* rue*)* is made from a plant whose taste is among the bitterest known, and is associated with acute aches and pains, cough, headache, hip pain and limitation of movement and stiffness. Associated mental and emotional symptoms include anxiety, depression, despair, dissatisfaction with self and others, lack of caring or emotional blunting and contradictory or quarrelsome disposition. Bending down, lying down, overexertion or prolonged sitting will worsen symptoms, as will nighttime and cold damp weather. Allergies, arthritis (especially osteo), asthma, back pain (especially sciatica), carpal tunnel syndrome, colds, constipation, fibromyalgia, gout, headaches (especially those related to eye strain) and sprains and strains have been successfully treated.

Sepia *(cuttlefish ink sac)* is another remedy classically used for women's illnesses and symptoms. It is helpful for chronic mucus production and congestion, cough, exhaustion and fatigue, fever, menstrual pain, nausea during pregnancy, joint and muscle stiffness and stomach upset. Patients are often anxious and aggressive, and may be bitter and critical; depression and feelings of disappointment are frequent, and forgetfulness may be combined with indifference, irritability and an independent streak. Scolding and bossy are other characteristics, along with jitteriness, rudeness and tearfulness. These are worsened by cold and damp weather and by storms, as well as exertion in heat or confinement to stuffy rooms. Walking, noises and being jarred or jostled are also aggravating factors. This has been used for anemia, back pain, bronchitis, chemotherapy-related symptoms, chronic fatigue, constipation, cystitis and urinary tract infections, depression, digestive disorders, dizziness, endometriosis, headaches (especially migraine with nausea), irritable bowel syndrome, menopausal and premenstrual or menstrual symptoms, morning sickness or miscarriage during pregnancy, ulcers, vaginitis and varicose veins.

Silicea (silica) in homeopathic doses causes chills, congestion and chronic phlegm production, fever, skin pimples,, decreased stamina, sour-smelling sweat and fatigue. Mental and emotional symptoms include anxiety, faintness of heart, fear of failure, frustration, homesickness, obstinacy, self-doubt and spitefulness. Bathing, damp drafts, stuffy rooms, wet weather, morning hours and being uncovered aggravate symptoms, as does hot food. This remedy causes the expulsion of foreign bodies such as splinters, and has been used for acne, allergies, anemia, bronchitis, carpal tunnel syndrome, cataracts, chronic fatigue, constipation, diabetes, diarrhea, digestive disorders, dizziness, earaches and ear infections, various other infections, insomnia, rheumatoid arthritis, and temporomandibular joint dysfunction. Right-sided symptoms are particularly benefitted.

Spomgiatosta (roasted sponge) is associated with dry or hacking cough, exhaustion, hoarseness and sore throat physically and anxiety, fear of dying and tearfulness emotionally. Symptoms are worse at midnight, and are aggravated by movement, sweating and being touched. Asthma, chronic fatigue, and colds and flu have benefitted from its use.

Staphysagria (stavesacre or lousewort) is used for depression, nausea, urinary disorders and the effects of various injuries. Patients are often abusive, irritable and in internal turmoil, tending to lash out verbally and sometimes physically; long-standing anger, resentment and suppressed grief are often associated. Cold temperatures and cold drinks, dehydration, menses, sleep deprivation; exposure to smoke and being touched are aggravating factors. The remedy has been prescribed for depression, eczema, headache, menopause and menstrual disorders, psoriasis and urinary tract disorders (bladder infections, cystitis, prostatic hypertrophy).

Sulphur was first studied by Hahnemann, and produced cough, diarrhea, exhaustion, fever, indigestion, itching and burning skin, muscle cramps, sore throat and the "sulphur mask", a patch of red skin over the nose from one cheek to the other. Patients are often anxious but careless and unkempt, sometimes selfish and desiring to be the center of attention, needing constant excitement and fearing boredom. The skin often appears unhealthy or even unclean and the scalp is dry. Alcohol use, bathing, nose blowing, coughing, being immobile, exposure to the open air or sunlight, and swallowing or talking worsen symptoms, and there is often an "11 a.m. slump". Many conditions have been treated with some success with *sulphur*: acne, alcoholism, anxiety, arthritis, asthma, back pain, bronchitis, chronic fatigue, constipation, diabetes, diarrhea, dizziness, earaches and ear infections, eczema, fibromyalgia, food allergies, influenza, hay fever, headache (especially migraine), hemorrhoids, hypoglycemia, indigestion, insomnia, irritable bowel syndrome, menopause and menstrual disorders, multiple sclerosis, complications of pregnancy, psoriasis, rheumatoid arthritis, ulcers and vaginitis.

Syzygium Jambolanum (jambol seed) is derived from the otherwise poisonous seeds of the rose apple tree *(Syzygium Jambos)*, and is reported in Indian studies to markedly reduce elevated blood sugar, even to the point of precipitating hypoglycemia. It is usually given in low potencies, such as the mother tincture of 3x or 6x dilution, and is taken before meals in order to reduce spikes of blood sugar with eating. It is particularly effective for patients with acute diabetic symptoms, like thirst, urinary frequency and weakness.

Tabacum (tobacco) is associated with chills and cold sweat, clammy skin, nausea and vomiting, pallor and stomach upset, and patients often feel anxious and giddy. Temperature extremes, stuffy rooms, movement and physical exertion are aggravating factors. Anxiety, dizziness, morning sickness in pregnancy and motion sickness otherwise are clinical indications.

Tarentula (Tarentula Hispanica, wolf spider) is the name generally applied to about 900 species of hairy spiders in the Old and New Worlds. Some are larger and more poisonous than others, but most are harmless and can be kept as pets. The Spanish or wolf spider is actually named for the Italian port of Taranto, and was long thought to be dangerous and to require rapid dancing (the *tarantella*) in order to escape trembling and mania after being bitten. In fact, wolf spiders are less dangerous than the unrelated larger tarantulas of South America, but do have venom, and the homeopathic remedy is produced with this. It is associated with restlessness, agitation, hyperactive senses, stabbing headache, rapid heartbeat and palpitations, often with shortness of breath and suffocation, craving for salty and highly seasoned foods but also for sand and aversion to meat, sexual excitability but worse symptoms after sex, skin fragility with breakdown and infection and sharp and shooting pain in the extremities. It may therefore be useful for the neuropathy and skin changes of diabetes if accompanied by some of these features.

Uranium Nitricum (uranium nitrate) is principally used for diabetes treatment, because profuse urination, urinary incontinence, glucose in the urine and frank diabetes have been produced by its administration. Dull and heavy pain, sore nose with acrid nasal discharge, eye inflammation, styes on the eyelids, urethral burning and bladder pain when full, excessive thirst and increased appetite with swollen abdomen but marked wasting and weight loss, boring or burning abdominal pain and sometimes ulcers, male impotence, cold and sweaty limbs and depression have also been described.

Urtica Urens (stinging nettle*)* is used for blotchy skin, fatigue, fever, itching and burning skin, joint pain and sore throat. It has no particular associated psychological symptoms, but physical manifestations are more marked after bathing or in the heat, when lying on the right side, after physical overexertion and in damp, cold or snowy weather. It has been used for allergic reactions and hives, cystitis, fibromyalgia, gout, injuries (particularly puncture wounds), insect bites, kidney stones, rheumatoid arthritis, shingles and vaginitis.

Vanadium Metallicum (vanadium) is used as a nutritional supplement for diabetes, as described below. As an oxygen carrier and catalyst of chemical reactions, homeopathic vanadium is used for many diseases involving wasting and emaciation but particularly for advanced or severe diabetes. Loss of appetite, thirst and increased drinking, protein and glucose in the urine (sometimes blood), large amounts of urine, weakness and wasting are the chief associated symptoms, and patients are often melancholy or hysterical and frequently have dizziness and vertigo. Retinal inflammation and visual loss, dry and irritated cough, anemia, fat infiltration of the liver and accelerated atherosclerosis of the heart, brain and peripheral blood vessels are also produced.

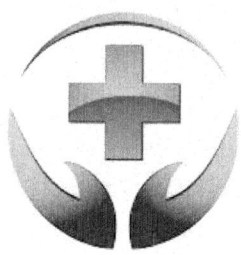

CHAPTER 7

CONSTITUTIONAL HOMEOPATHIC MEDICINE

In the slightly more than 200 years since homeopathic remedies began to be used, profiles of physical, mental and emotional characteristics have been developed that may predict which of these medications are likely to help a particular patient. The correct remedy selected according to an individual's "constitution" will normalize energy, improve overall health and thereby effect improvement in a chronic illness, whether diabetes or arthritis or headaches. The remedy or remedies suggested by a particular profile are usually taken twice a day in 30x, 12c or 30c potencies for one or two weeks, and then changed to something else of symptoms persist or stopped if there has been improvement and tried again later if the underlying condition deteriorates.

The constitutional profile of *Calcarea Carbonica* is plumpness or obesity, easy fatigability, susceptibility to infections, especially of the ear or upper respiratory tract and chilliness. Children are often delayed in development. There is profuse sweating, especially during sleep and particularly on the neck and back of the head, and patients often have brittle nails that break easily. Chronic constipation and a tendency to crave eggs, dairy products and sweets may be present. Mental and emotional features include being work-oriented and organized, independent, curious and stubborn, but prone to worry and easily overwhelmed by difficulties.

Those who may respond to *Lycopodium* often have digestive symptoms such as gas and bloating, which worsen between 4 and 8 p.m. Respiratory illnesses are also present, and symptoms often predominate on the right side. Their appetites are often large and they crave sweets. They may also be domineering but have low self-esteem.

People responsive to *Syzygium Jambos* often have headaches, sometimes severe, and are worse between 10 a.m. and 3 p.m. They also have cold sores and marked eye and skin sensitivity to the sun. Depression and past bereavement are frequent, but they do not like to cry in front of others, and are famously neat and tidy. They often prefer to be alone, and often have a craving for salty foods.

Phosphorus types are prone to respiratory infections and often have asthma. Nosebleeds are also frequent, as are digestive upsets, and they often crave sweets and ice cream and want cold drinks. This is associated with an outgoing personality, sociability, empathy for others and a desire for attention; they often do not like to be alone, especially in the dark.

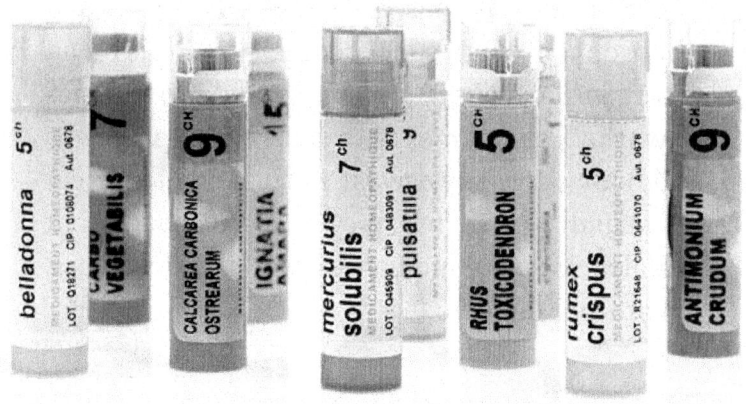

People who will benefit from *Pulsatilla*, more often women and children, are easily overheated and prefer to be in the fresh air. They crave sweets but are generally not thirsty, and are prone to sinusitis and ear or respiratory infections, often with yellow-green discharges.

They are often shy and easily hurt, but at the same time crave attention.

The constitution benefitted by *Silicea* is susceptible to infections and has reduced stamina. This is often associated with low weight and brittle hair and nails and fragile skin, as well as chilliness and cold sensitivity. Irritability and stubbornness is often combined with shyness and sensitivity.

The *Sulphur* type has been labeled "the ragged philosopher", and such people are messy and disorganized, often unkempt and sometimes unwashed, sometimes with severe skin problems and body odor. They sweat easily, and have great thirst and appetite for spicy food and sweets, but are also sociable, inquisitive and like to discuss, debate and theorize.

The Cell Salts and Their Uses

The German homeopathic physician Wilhelm Schüssler showed in the 1870s that deficient or unbalanced mineral levels in cells were involved in a number of diseases, and developed for these 12 homeopathic remedies that he called "biochemic cell salts. These compounds have been widely used to restore mineral deficiencies and enhance energy metabolism in chronic diseases, thereby facilitating conventional or homeopathic medical treatment and minimizing complications. The salts are available in tablet, pellet or liquid form, usually at a potency of 6x, and it is recommended to take 1 or 2 between meals for chronic conditions, or 1 every 15 to 60 minutes for acute problems. Tablets can be crushed and mixed with an ounce of purified water, and then administered to children with a dropper or teaspoon.

Calcarea fluorica (calcium fluoride)

strengthens connective tissue, and is used for ligament and tendon improves bone health, and is used to enhance healing of fractures, prevent osteoporosis, manage teething and alleviate growing pains. *Calcarea Sulphurica* (calcium sulfate) assists with healing, and is used for abscesses, boils and skin eruptions like acne.

Ferrum phosphoricum (iron phosphate)

is similar to the iron preparations of conventional medicine, and is used for anemia and the consequences of profuse bleeding, as well as to alleviate the exhaustion that can attend chronic illnesses and fevers. *Magnesia phosphoric* (magnesium phosphate) is effective for muscle and nerve disorders, particularly muscle cramps, spasmodic stomach pain, seizures and nervous system hyperactivity. *Silicea* (silica), described above, is also a tissue cleanser, effective for acne, skin lesions discharging pus and chronic respiratory and sinus infections.

Potassium and sodium are the chief bases of the cell salts. *Kali muriaticum* (potassium chloride) decreases mucus production, and is useful for ear, sinus and throat infections with pain and drainage. *Kali phospohricum* (potassium phosphate) is particularly effective in nerve stabilization, and is used as to enhance attention and decrease anxiety, as well as for pain after nerve injury.

Kali sulphuricum (potassium sulfate) works primarily on the skin, and heals and dries draining or infected skin areas. *Natrum Muriaticum* (sodium chloride) adjusts water balance in tissues, and is used for dry skin and mucous membranes, cold sores, hay fever and also for the physical and psychological symptoms of grief. *Natrum Phosphoricum* (sodium phosphate) is involved in acid-base balance, and has been used for heartburn and vaginitis due to bacterial or fungal overgrowth that is stimulated by abnormal tissue acidity there. *Natrum Sulphuricum* (sodium sulfate) aids detoxification, and is effective for colitis, head injury, hepatitis and jaundice of the newborn.

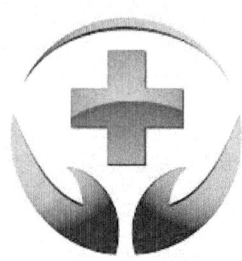

CHAPTER 8

HOMEOPATHIC TREATMENT OF COMMON DISORDERS

There is extensive literature and clinical experience regarding the use of most of the above medications for various disorders. In contrast to allopathic medicine, in which the focus is usually on identifying a disease for which a particular medication or group of medicines is indicated, the focus in homeopathic practice is usually on identifying a particular symptom or group of symptoms that are likely to respond to a particular medication (keynotes) or on identifying particular characteristics of the patient that in past experience have predicted response to one or another medication (remedy profiles). Nevertheless, most common conditions have over the years become associated with certain remedies that may be the most appropriate to try first. Many of these are summarized below, but in the event of minimal response to the most commonly used medications or some adverse effect or aggravation of symptoms by an apparently appropriate remedy, the advice of a homeopathic physician is invaluable.

Abscesses are the accumulation of pus on or under the skin, or inside tissues and organs; an abscess under the surface of the skin is a *carbuncle* and one involving a hair follicle is usually termed a *boil*. These are painful and can reach a large size or spread, particularly in association with underlying diseases or compromised immune function. Incision and drainage and sometimes surgical drainage followed by antibiotics are generally required. **Belladonna** may be an alternative for red, swollen or throbbing lesions, associated with fever but often without pus. **Hepar Sulphuris** is recommended for tender and painful abscesses that have come to a head, with pus that can be seen or smelled, and the remedy in fact speeds the opening and drainage of the abscess or boil and the evacuation of pus. **Lachesis** has been recommended for dark blue or purple boils with pustules and pain or tenderness, especially on the left side. **Mercurius Solubilis** is also used for dark-colored pustules with pain and draining pus. **Silicea,** which for unknown reasons facilitates the expulsion of foreign material, may aid in the expression of pus.

Acne represents the accumulation of sebum, the oily lubricant of the skin, along with blocked pores and bacterial or yeast overgrowth and skin inflammation, and is often managed with recurrent doses of antibiotics, topical lotions or vitamin A derivatives, all of which can lead to complications. Homeopathic options include **Calcarea Carbonica** for acne with yellowish discharge, **Hepar Sulphuricum** for tender pus-filled spots or **Ledum** for pustular acne on the nose and cheeks that is improved by cold applications. **Pulsatilla** is effective for acne in women that is affected by hormonal changes. **Silicea** has been used for persistent white pustules, while **Sulphur** helps sore or itchy pustules or those that are worsened by washing.

Allergies often produce watering and burning of the eyes, nasal discharge and sneezing, and **Allium cepa** is effective for these. **Arsenicum album** often works for sensitive and fastidious people with multiple allergies, particularly when the nose as well as the eyes burns and is irritated by the discharge. **Euphrasia** or "eyebright" has long been used for red and irritated eyes. **Histaminium** is made specifically for allergy treatment from histadines, plant compounds that mimic the allergic effects of histamine, and alleviates nasal and respiratory symptoms that come on very rapidly.

Lycopodium has been used for right-sided nasal congestion and sore throat, often with indigestion after meals. **Natrum Muriaticum** works best for nasal congestion and sneezing triggered by sun exposure, often associated with cold sores and frequently with craving for salty foods. People who awaken with sneezing and congestion and who crave sweets, alcohol or tobacco may respond best to **Nux vomica**, principally men, while women or children may be more likely to respond to **Pulsatilla**, especially if allergies are worse in warm rooms or at night and are relieved by fresh air. **Silicea** particularly helps upper airway symptoms such as wheezing, and works for people who have reduced stamina and frequent infections.

Alzheimer's Disease

Alzheimer's Disease - The mood and behavioral symptoms of *Alzheimer's disease* and some other forms of dementia may be helped by **Alumina**, the homeopathic dilution of aluminum, especially if confusion and memory problems are associated with constipation. **Helleborus Niger**, **Lycopodium**, **Plumbum**and **Sulphur** have also been used for confusion, difficulty speaking and repeating, fearfulness, paranoia and agitated behavior.

Anemia takes many forms and has a variety of causes. Iron deficiency is the leading cause, and iron utilization is improved by **Ferrumphos Phoricum**. **Calcarea Phosphorica** has helped anemia in children and the anemia resulting from blood loss or chronic diseases in adults, which have also been helped by **China**. **Natrum Muriaticum**has been recommended for anemia accompanied by headache or constipation.

Anxiety refers to a variety of disorders involving dread of specific events or outcomes, fear of unspecified bad things that may happen and physical manifestations of panic or terror. These are often associated with depression, and may have a familial basis. Panic attacks are often managed with **Aconite**, while fear and insecurity are often treated with **Arsenicum album**, especially in people with obsessions or compulsions. **Calcarea Carbonica** is used for anxiety associated with exhaustion, fatigue and a feeling of being overwhelmed. **Gelsemium** is effective for anxiety with physical symptoms such as diarrhea or tremor, and has been used for performance anxiety such as stage fright. **Ignatia** is effective for anxiety that is accompanied by anger, resentment and rumination, and many people who respond to it have *globushystericus*, a persistent feeling that there is a lump in their throat. **Kali phosphoricum** is used for free-floating anxiety, especially with fatigue and memory problems.

Performance anxiety and anxiety in social situations like meeting strangers and being in large groups are often helped by **Lycopodium.**

Arthritis is usually a manifestation of rheumatoid arthritis or some related immune disorder or due to osteoarthritis, the degenerative deterioration of joints. Because homeopathy predates this differentiation, the same remedies are usually used for both types, although osteoarthritis is the predominant problem treated homeopathically. **Apis** is more often used for rheumatoid arthritis, with joints that resemble a bee sting, hot and swollen and with stinging pain, often relieved by the application of cold. **Arnica** may be used for both types, but particularly when there is associated bruising or the joints are sore and feel bruised. **Belladonna** also helps red, swollen and hot joints, especially of sudden onset. People who are irritable, worse with any attempt at movement and do not want to move swollen and painful joints may improve with **Bryonia.** **Calcarea Carbonica** helps joint pain worsened by cold and damp, and works best for people who are overweight and often feel cold. **Calcarea Fluorica** is more effective for chronically swollen joints with bone spurs, while the arthritis improved by **Calcarea Phosphoric** is aggravated by cold air or drafts and is often confined to the neck or related to bone spurs. **Pulsatilla** is often used for "palindromic rheumatism", joint pain that moves from place to place and is sometimes a feature of fibromyalgia. Arthritis associated with stiffness, improved by movement and warmth and worsened by cold, damp and periods of inactivity may be helped particularly by **Rhus Toxicodendron. Sulphur** is recommended for arthritis associated with burning pain, often improved by cold applications.

Asthma has been treated with many homeopathic medicines, but emergent conventional treatment is needed for acute episodes of respiratory distress. **Aconite** is nevertheless used for acute episodes, particularly those precipitated by exposure to cold air and associated with fright and anxiety. **Arsenicum album** is often used for asthma that is worse between midnight and 2 a.m., worsened by cold air and improved by sitting up and attended by anxiety and restlessness. **Carbo Vegetabilis** has been used for chilly patients who feel faint and are improved by sitting near a window or being fanned; asthma is often associated with gas and abdominal fullness, and patients feel worse for eating, lying down or talking. Asthma accompanied by copious mucus with coughing or gagging may respond to

Ipecacuanha. When asthma worsens between 2 and 4 a.m. or is improved by sitting up and leaning forward, this may be an indication for **Kali carbonicum. Lachesis** is effective for asthma with throat and chest constriction and inability to tolerate being touched in these areas; people feel hot and are improved by fresh air. **Natrum Sulphuricum** is recommended for asthma worse in the early morning and precipitated or worsened by cold damp air. **Nux vomica** works for people who are chilly, irritable, overindulge in spicy food or alcohol and may have gastrointestinal symptoms along with asthma. **Pulsatilla** is often used for asthma in women or when comfort or attention is needed; fresh air is also desired, and symptoms are often worse in hot stuffy rooms or after eating fatty food; there is often thick yellow mucus.

Attention Deficit Hyperactivity Disorder is now known to persist into adulthood and to have pervasive adverse effect on education, social adjustment and occupational success. Conventional treatment is mostly focused on stimulants that are controlled substances, and there is worry that these may interfere with growth. Several benign homeopathic alternatives are frequently used, some of them among the more obscure remedies. **Sulphur** has been used in children who are

hyperactive, curious and stubborn, often with heat, thirst, profuse sweating and desire for spicy foods and cold drinks. **Tarentula** helps restless, impulsive children who are sometimes impulsive and destructive, and are fond of music and dancing. Less common remedies used for ADHD include **Anacardium Orientale**, made from the Indian marking nut tree and helpful for absent-mindedness and forgetfulness, as well as **Hyoscyamus Niger,** from the otherwise poisonous nightshade henbane, which has been used for impulsive, violent and talkative behavior. **Medorrhinum** is a "nosode", a remedy prepared directly from diseased tissue, in this case the sterilized and highly diluted pus from the skin pustules of gonorrhea: it is used for violent behavior and temper tantrums. **Stramonium** (thornapple) helps children with nighttime fears and night terrors and anger and rage during the day. **Tuberculinum** is another nosode, made from the sputum of tuberculosis patients, but when sterilized and diluted is a safe remedy for stubborn, demanding and impulsive children who may manifest violent behavior and cruelty toward animals.

Back pain is one of the most common complaints in primary-care physician visits, and is in most series the leading cause of neurological and neurosurgical referral. The cost and complications of back surgery and growing concern about the overuse and misuse of prescription pain medications makes alternative medical solutions very attractive. **Aesculus Hippocastum** (horse chestnut) is sometimes used for back pain that radiates into the hips and is worse in the sitting position. **Arnica** is widely used for back pain as for other painful complaints, particularly after injury and with limitation of motion by pain. **Bryonia** is effective for pain that is worse with attempts at movement and that is accompanied by stiffness and worsened by cold. **Calcarea Carbonica** also works for back pain that is worse in cold, and in people who tend to feel cold. **Cimcifuga Racemosa** (black cohosh) has long been used in Native American and European herbalism for menstrual cramps and related symptoms, and works as well for back pain with stiffness and soreness. **Ignatia** has been recommended for back pain aggravated by anger, grief or emotional upset, while **Magnesia phosphoric** helps more straightforward back pain after injury or exertion that is accompanied by muscle spasm. **Nux vomica** is often used for back pain accompanied by constipation and headache, often with irritability and a tendency to overindulge in food and drink. **Rhus Toxicodendron** is a specific remedy for muscle strain or ligament sprain, and works for pain that is accompanied by restlessness, worse with immobility and better with movement and aggravated by cold and dampness. **Ruta** is often used for neck and shoulder pain, less frequently for the lower back, and is indicated when arms or legs feel weak or lame and pain is worse at night.

Bone fractures require conventional medical evaluation and usually orthopedic treatment, but the speed of healing and associated complications may be improved by homeopathic remedies. **Aconite** helps with acute shock and pain after injury, often followed by **Arnica** for the swelling and bruising that may accompany a fracture. **Bryonia**, which helps people immobilized by pain who do not want to move a limb, or in the case of healing fracture should not move it, is often used thereafter. **Calcarea Carbonica** is useful when fractures occur as a result of brittle bones, as with osteoporosis, and has been shown to be effective for pain and various other symptoms in people who are flabby, feel chilly and are worse when they are cold. The closely related **Calcarea Phosphoric** stimulates the formation of new bone and may help slowly healing fractures. Injuries that cause fractures may cause nerve injury as well, particularly crush injuries, and some fractures, like that of the coccyx or tailbone, are often accompanied by persistent pain apparently due to nerve irritation; this is often improved by **Hypericum. Phosphorus** is also used for "pathological fractures" due to bone disease, and has been associated with therapeutic response in tall, thin people and those who are social, suggestible and very fond of ice-cold drinks. **Silicea** also helps when bone density is reduced, as in osteoporosis, and may be particularly useful in the elderly and those with chronic illnesses. **Symphytum** (*Symphytum officinale*) is an old herbal remedy widely believed to cause prompt bone healing, and may be the most common alternative therapy for fractures; the bone should be set and casted before Symphytum is given because of the speed with which fractures reunite thereafter.

Bronchitis is commonly treated with antibiotics and sometimes with other prescription drugs, and if chronic or recurrent can require repeated courses of these with the potential for side effects. Homeopathic options include **Antimonium Tartaricum** for congestion and wet cough but with difficulty producing sputum, often improved by cool surroundings, or **Arsenicum album** for cough with burning pain, anxiety and fatigue, and worsening between midnight and 2 a.m., often improved by warm drinks. **Bryonia** helps when coughing causes pain, reluctance to move and sometimes irritability and thirst. **Coccus cacti**, which is made from a dried and powdered Mexican insect (cochineal), is used for cough which produces tenacious mucus, while **Drosera Rotundifolia**, made from the carnivorous plant Sundew, helps dry hacking cough that is not productive. **Hepar Sulphuris** works on rattling and barking coughs with mucus production, particularly when exposed to cold or dry air and accompanied by coldness and irritability. **Kali bichromium** is also effective for productive cough, but more often one accompanied by hoarseness and worsened by eating and drinking. People who respond to **Phosphorus** report burning chest discomfort and have a dry tickling cough that is often worse when lying on the left side. In contrast, coughing suggestive of **Pulsatilla** response is worse when lying down on the back, is loose in the morning and dry later in the day and produces green or yellow phlegm. **Silicea** helps with recurrent or chronic cough, particularly in association with decreased stamina or immune compromise; expectoration of mucus is often difficult. **Spongia Tosta** works for dry and hacking cough that is improved by warm foods or drinks, while improvement with cold drinks and undue warmth and desire for cool surroundings may suggest **Sulphur**, particularly if bronchitis has been present for a long time or with burning chest pain.

Burns, whether thermal, chemical or sun-related, may respond to several homeopathic remedies but may need more specialized burn care if severe or widespread. **Apis** helps with burning, stinging, heat and skin puffiness. **Arsenicum album** helps burned skin that is worse in cold air and better with warmth, particularly with dark skin discoloration and often in anxious and restless people. The blistering that can follow burns is antagonized with a remedy made from the blister beetle, **Cantharis vesicatoria**, and this is particularly helpful for intense sunburn, scalding and second- or third-degree burns, especially if cold water alleviates some of their pain. **Causticum** (potassium hydrate) was first prepared by Hahnemann himself by burning potash and lime derived from marble; it is a highly caustic substance but in homeopathic dilution works safely on burns from caustic chemicals, as well as poorly-healing burns of other cause. **Hypericum**, mentioned earlier for nerve injuries, is effective for burns that are followed by neuropathic or nerve pain, while **Phosphorus** works particularly on the burning and shooting pain that can follow electrical burns. **Rhus Toxicodendron** is helpful for burning or itching pain accompanied by skin blistering or vesicles, often with restlessness and improvement by the application of hot water and worsening by cold water. **Urticaurens** can be used along with Cantharis for burning pain with blistering, more often for first-degree burns.

Cancer - Homeopathic remedies have little role in the treatment of *cancer*, but some are helpful for preventing or reducing the adverse effects of chemotherapy or radiation. **Cadmium Suphuratum** is prepared from the generally toxic metal cadmium, and is little used today but contributed to the beneficial effects shown with homeopathic treatment in cholera and yellow fever outbreaks of the 19th century; with toxicity removed by repeated dilution, this remedy reduces fatigue and nausea or vomiting and may prevent hair loss during cancer treatment. **Ipecacuanha** is effective for nausea and vomiting, and **Nux Vomica** may prevent diarrhea, constipation, heartburn, nausea and other gastrointestinal side effects.

Cardiovascular disease likewise requires conventional medical evaluation and therapy, particularly for acute symptoms, although natural medicine preparations may help to retard some of the precipitating causes of heart disease like hypertension and elevated cholesterol. **Aconite** may help at the onset of the chest pain and other symptoms of angina pectoris, and **Arnica** may help with squeezing chest pain or the feeling of being bruised. **Cactus**, made from the cactus plant *Cereus grandiflora*, has been used for angina, particularly band-like chest tightening. These are only for symptomatic relief, however.

Carpal tunnel syndrome is one of the

most common peripheral nerve injuries, and may affect 10 per cent or more of the growing number of people who work at computers. Conventional therapy with corticosteroid injection or surgical decompression of the median nerve is not always optimal, and often cannot be done at an early stage although symptoms may be uncomfortable. **Arnica** is effective for early nerve injury in the first few days after the onset of symptoms, while **Causticum** can help in long lasting carpal tunnel syndrome, with burning pain, wrist stiffness and contracture of the wrist. The pain results from nerve injury, so **Hypericum** is often effective. **Rhus Toxicodendron** helps persistent wrist aching and numbness that is sometimes alleviated by shaking the hand or otherwise moving, as does **Ruta** if the hand feels stiff or weak.

Cataracts are usually dealt with surgically,

but their formation and progression may be slowed by homeopathic treatments. **Calcarea**

Carbonica has been found to slow the progression of cataracts without visual symptoms, while **Phosphorus** may be effective at the early stages of visual clouding. Decreased vision with redness or heat in and around the eyes may respond to **Ruta**, and **Silicea** has been reported to alleviate dimming of vision with more advanced cataracts.

Chronic Fatigue Syndrome is a
common cause for alternative medicine consultation, usually because a specific diagnosis has not been found in conventional medical evaluation and medical treatments, sometimes many of them, have been ineffective. Exhaustion, depression and anxiety are common symptoms and often respond to **Arsenicum album**, especially when insomnia, chilliness and worsening of symptoms by cold are also present. People prone to fatigue and anxiety or who tend to take on too much may have less fatigue with **Calcarea Carbonica**, especially if they are mildly overweight and sweat readily. **Gelsemium** is often used for physical fatigue with drowsiness, weakness and muscle pain, while mental fatigue may respond to **Kali phosphoricum**. **Phosphoric acid**, a common ingredient in carbonated soft drinks, helps fatigue attended by the craving for such drinks or in the aftermath of grief. People with chronic fatigue, minimal

exercise tolerance and susceptibility to infections may respond to **Silicea**.

Colds are still little helped by conventional medical treatment, but may be alleviated by **Oscillococcinum**, a French remedy prepared from the liver and heart of Barbary ducks (*Anas Barbariae Hepatis et cordis*), which is the best-selling over-the-counter medication in Europe. **Aconite** also shortens the duration and reduces the severity of cold symptoms if taken within 4 hours of onset. **Allium cepa** helps with burning eyes and nasal discharge that irritates the upper lip and nostrils, while similar discharges that do not burn suggest the use of **Arsenicum album**. **Ferrum Phosphoricum** helps people who are feverish but have no other symptoms, while **Gelsemium** is more effective for aching, chills, fatigue or headache. Colds that come on in hot or cold weather and are attended by coated tongue, sore throat and increased salivation may respond to **Mercurius Solubilis**, while colds attended by sneezing and clear nasal discharge or with cold sores will improve with **Natrum Muriaticum. Nux vomica** is often given for colds characterized by chilliness, irritability, congestion, coughing, sneezing and sore throat, while **Pulsatilla** decreases green or yellow nasal mucus and lessens congestion, especially in people who want to be in fresh air and to be comforted.

Constipation is the most common gastrointestinal disorder in developed countries, and is frequently due to excessive dietary fat and insufficient dietary fiber and fluids. Laxatives are sometimes needed, but overuse of either over-the-counter laxatives or prescription drugs to stimulate bowel function may cause more problems than they solve. **Alumina** helps with infrequent very hard stools, especially if attended by memory problems and **Bryonia** is effective when hard stools are attended by headache, irritability and thirst. People who respond to **Calcarea Carbonica** are usually constipated, feel tired or overwhelmed and are flabby and have sweaty hands and feet. **Lycopodium** works for constipation alternating with bloating and flatulence, usually worse in the afternoon and better after warm beverages. **Natrum Muriaticum** helps constipation in people who have photosensitivity and may be depressed, and also with thirst and craving for salt. Chronic constipation is one of the keynotes for **Nux vomica**, usually attended by headache and irritability, overwork and undue exercise, overindulgence in food and drink and past overuse of laxatives. Women with menstrual cramps, premenstrual syndrome or menopausal symptoms may respond to **Sepia**, particularly if they have persistent abdominal and rectal heaviness. Bowel movements that come out partially and then recede, and that require frequent straining, may warrant the use of **Silicea**, and constipation alternating with diarrhea or with rectal pain and burning may respond to **Sulphur.**

Cough is a very common but nonspecific symptom, and needs evaluation if persistent for more than two weeks or accompanied by bloody or obviously infected sputum or by breathing difficulty. If benign, nagging coughs may improve with the homeopathic remedies discussed earlier in connection with "Bronchitis".

Crohn's Disease or regional ileitis is an inflammatory and possibly autoimmune condition in which the small intestine, less frequently the large intestine and occasionally other parts of the digestive tract develop ulcerations and then scarring. Corticosteroids and drugs that suppress the immune system are the mainstay of therapy, and can lead to significant complications, but the course of the disease can be beneficially affected by holistic interventions. **Arsenicum album** is particularly effective for burning abdominal pain, often attended by restlessness and anxiety. Throbbing or burning abdominal pain of sudden onset with fever suggests the use of **Belladonna. Colocynth** is helps sharp and colicky abdominal pain, while abdominal pain associated with emotional upset, grief or resentment may respond to **Ignatia. Magnesia phosphoric** helps abdominal cramping that is aggravated by pressure, and **Nux vomica** works for pain of this type in people who are chilly, irritable and have headaches. Pain associated with diarrhea, especially triggered by rich foods or occurring at night, may be helped by **Pulsatilla**. Burning pain and diarrhea during the night may respond to **Sulphur**.

Dementia is the loss over a period of 6 months of more of cognitive abilities that were formerly present. There are a variety of causes for this, ranging from Alzheimer's disease and its variants to the effects of multiple strokes, syphilis involving the nervous system (now rare), vitamin deficiency, medication effects and depression or dehydration. Medical and neurologic evaluation is necessary, but conventional medical treatment is still limited in its effectiveness. **Alumina**, the homeopathic dilution of powdered aluminum, can lessen confusion and improve memory, particularly in those who are also constipated. People who are flabby, chilly and perspire easily on the head, neck and feet may have improvement in attention span, less confusion, reduction in behavior problems and less difficulty in verbal recall with **Calcarea Carbonica**. Poor memory attended by mental fatigue may be helped by **Kali phosphoricum**, while **Lycopodium** may work for memory problems that are attended by gastrointestinal symptoms. **Sulphur** works for people who have difficulty naming and whose recall is poor early in the day but then improves, often associated with being hot and craving cold drinks and spicy food.

Depression affects more than 10 per cent of the population, women more than men, and there is continuing concern about the long-term effects of even newer and more benign antidepressant drugs. While underlying medical and neurological causes need to be considered, and suicidal thoughts or gestures require emergent evaluation and treatment, depression of mild to moderate severity may be helped by homeopathic remedies. **Arsenicum album** helps depression in fastidious, perfectionistic and obsessive people, who may also have phobias, restlessness and insomnia between midnight and 2 a.m. Despair and suicidality with inability to feel pleasure but some improvement with sun exposure may be improved by **Aurum metallicum. Ignatia** is effective for depression

116

attended by chronic emotional upset, and rapid mood swings, frequent sighing a lump in the throat are prominent parts of the remedy profile. People who are mentally fatigued and depressed in mood on account of overwork may be helped by **Kali phosphoricum,** while depressed people who do not express emotions and are aggravated by the consolation of others often improve with **Natrum Muriaticum. Pulsatilla** is particularly helpful for depression in women, often associated with menstrual or menopausal symptoms and with sensitivity, a need for attention and reassurance and craving for sweets. Depressed women also respond preferentially to **Sepia**, particularly at menses or in menopause, but these tend to be irritable, disinterested in sex, disengaged from their families, chilly and very desirous of sweets and sour or salty food. **Staphysagria**, made from the stavesacre or lousewort plant, helps people with suppressed anger and resentment, reluctance to stand up for themselves, headaches and insomnia as well as depression.

Seasonal Affective Disorder - A

related condition involving the periodic recurrence of depressive symptoms in relation to the length of the day and the amount of ambient sunlight is *Seasonal Affective Disorder.* Depression and prominent complaints of desire for sleep, fatigue and difficulty concentrating usually arise in dark winter months and remit in the summer, although cycling in the reverse order can occur. In addition to antidepressant medications, treatment with intense fluorescent lights is often recommended, which may not always be convenient. In addition to the above remedies, **Aurum metallicum** may help deeply depressed people who have lost the ability to experience pleasure (anhedonia) or who have suicidal thoughts. Suicidality should always be evaluated professionally.

Diabetes - Most of the classical homeopathic remedies are not specifically indicated for *Diabetes*, and not even the most devoted follower of Hahnemann and his successors would suggest that these preparations should be used instead of insulin. The selection of homeopathic remedies is based on matching the patient's symptoms to the symptoms produced when healthy people take the substance from which the remedy is made, and none of the early proving gave rise to a case of diabetes mellitus. In addition, the diagnosis of diabetes is based in large part on laboratory measurements that were not available in Hahnemann's time and for some years afterward, so there is little evidence correlating these measurements with specific homeopathic remedies. Many of the symptoms and complaints that people with diabetes report do match the profiles of different homeopathic medicines, however, and it is on this basis that remedies can be chosen, to alleviate numbness, tingling, frequent urination or fatigue rather than to normalize blood sugar or reduce hemoglobin A1c, which is an indicator of the degree pf diabetic control. Remedies derived from acids are commonly used for diabetes, particularly for acute symptoms and complications.

Diabetes is frequently associated with acidosis, an increased acidity of blood or tissue due to an excess of hydrogen ions. Ketoacidosis, the most serious diabetic complication, ought according to homeopathic principles to be treated or prevented by the use of a similarly acid diluted remedy. These remedies include **Aceticum Acidum**, **Carbolicum Acidum**, **Phosphoricum Acidum**, **Lacticum Acidum**, **Nitricumacidum**, and **Picrinicum Acidum**. Remedies made from minerals may be more useful for longer-term diabetes treatment, possibly because certain metals in very small amounts are necessary for the chemical reactions by which insulin causes cells to take in sugar, and thereby regulates the blood sugar level. The metal-based remedies are **Argentum Metallicum** and **nitricum**, **Aurum Metallicum**, **Cuprum Metallicum**, **Plumbum Metallicum**, **Uranium Nitricum** and **Vanadium Metallicum**. Remedies of plant origin are less often used in Western homeopathic practice but are often useful adjuncts to conventional treatment to improve control of blood sugar or to reduce the symptoms of neuropathy, retinopathy or peripheral vascular disease. These include **Nux vomica, Cephalandra Indica, Chionanthus, Chimaphilla, China, Curara, Helleborus Niger,** and **Syzygium Jambolanum.** Animal-derived remedies are sometimes prescribed as well, usually to improve whatever symptoms diabetic patients report based on their individual constitutions; these include **Lachesis, Crotalushorridus, Lac defloratum, Moschus** and **Tarentula.**

Diarrhea is along with constipation among the most common digestive problems. **Aloe,** widely used for skin care and in herbal medicine, is helpful for diarrhea with loud bowel sounds and yellowish, mucus-filled stools. **Argentum nitricum** has been used for diarrhea related to anxiety or anticipation, or caused by excessive sugar intake. **Arsenicum album** is effective for food poisoning, other types of diarrhea associated with vomiting and diarrhea with blood in the stool; people who respond are often fastidious, anxious and sensitive to cold, and warm drinks may improve symptoms. **Chamomilla** is useful for diarrhea in infants, which is often green or yellow and often accompanies teething. **China**, initially used for malaria, is also helpful for extreme diarrhea that causes exhaustion and weakness, while **Ipecacuanha** helps diarrhea that is attended by nausea.

Protracted watery stools may indicate the use of **Phosphorus**, while explosive but painless diarrhea that is worse in the morning may call for **Podophyllum. Pulsatilla** works for diarrhea after eating fruit or fatty foods, while explosive morning diarrhea with a sulfurous rotten-egg smell and irritation of the anus and rectum is often helped by **Sulphur**. When diarrhea is painful and very watery, it may respond to **Veratrum album**, made from the white hellebore plant.

Dizziness and *vertigo* are sometimes used interchangeably, but the former term really refers to unsteadiness, lack of equilibrium or faintness, while the latter indicates the sensation of spinning or the feeling that the environment is rotating. Dizziness can arise from many neurological, cardiac and psychological causes or from the effects of medication, while vertigo is generally produced by disorders of the inner ear and parts of the central nervous system. Some of the same homeopathic remedies are used for both kinds of imbalance, and there are several

121

commercial combination preparations available. **Aconite** is helpful for sudden attacks of dizziness associated with anxiety, panic or shock, sometimes with rapid pulse and fear that unconsciousness or even death may soon occur. **Bryonia** is used for dizziness when arising from sitting or with head turning or bending over, especially if irritability and thirst for cold drinks are also present. **Cocculus** has long been used for motion sickness with dizziness, anxiety or nausea and vomiting. Dizziness with lying down, turning the head or moving the head or eyes may respond to **Conium maculatum**. Dizziness attended by anxiety and particularly stage fright has been treated with **Gelsemium**, which also helps with dizziness and vertigo due to viral infections. **Nux vomica** is often used for dizziness from hangover or after overeating, and for food poisoning, which may produce dizziness. **Pulsatilla** often helps dizziness in women, or dizziness in warm and stuffy rooms, which is worse when lying down and better in the open air.

Earaches and ear infections can also

be treated with commercially available homeopathic combinations, with different preparations for adults and children. **Aconite** often helps earache or sudden onset, with restlessness and thirst, often worse in cold and dry wind and associated with bright red ears; this remedy will generally work only if used within a few hours of symptom onset. **Belladonna** helps hot, red, painful ears, which are throbbing and are associated with fever and dilated pupils; the right ear is more often or more severely affected than the left, and the eardrum is often red also. **Chamomilla** is used for irritable, crying, agitated children with severe earache, who often want to be carried but are calmed for only short periods by being held. Such earaches are often associated with teething, and children will often have one red cheek and one pale cheek. **Ferrumphos Phoricum** works especially well for children with fever who feel warm and have a red face and ear but do not otherwise appear very sick, in contrast to the acutely ill appearance that may suggest Belladonna. **Hepar Sulphuricus** is indicated for ears that are very tender and sensitive to cold and touch; children are often very irritable and have sharp ear pain ameliorated by the application of warmth, as well as pus or clear discharge from the ear. **Lachesis** always works best on left-sided symptoms, and earaches and infections are no exception; earache may in time move to the right ear and is worse at night and with warmth. Right-sided ear pain in contrast responds to **Lycopodium**, especially if accompanied by irritability, gas and flatulence, better with warm applications and worse between 4 and 8 p.m. When there is much pus or a malodorous discharge as well as sweatiness, **Mercurius** may help, particularly if there is also a coated tongue, increased salivation and bad breath, all worse at night. Children with earache who are weepy and want to be held and comforted may respond to **Pulsatilla**, and will also be worse at night and in warmth but better in open air and when cold is applied to the ear, and may also have yellow-green nasal and ear discharge. **Silicea** helps people with earache, especially children, who are thin, frail and prone to chronic infections. It is also used for acute infections when the eardrum is ruptured.

Eating disorder, principally anorexia nervosa and bulimia, can be life disrupting or even life-threatening and often require extensive endocrine evaluation and sometimes protracted psychiatric treatment. Homeopathic remedies may be less complicated to use than standard psychiatric drugs, particularly **Ferrum Phosphoricum** for iron deficiency and anemia. **Ignatia** helps people with mood swings, emotional upset and particularly grief and the chronic sensation of a lump in the throat, which psychoanalysts used to call "globushystericus" although the people, mainly women, who experience this are usually not hysterical. **Lycopodium** helps with eating problems accompanied by stomach upset, gas and bloating, hypoglycemia, irritability and low self-esteem. **Natrum Muriaticum** will help people who are depressed or have long-standing grief, as well as those who are sensitive to the sun, chronically thirsty and crave salty foods. Sensitive, weepy people who feel better with company, have a sweet tooth and prefer to be in cool air will often respond to **Pulsatilla.**

Eczema, or allergy-mediated inflammation of the skin with an accompanying rash, is among the most common skin disorders and affects about 10 per cent of the population. Homeopathic combination remedies are available, which contain in very small dose several compounds that have been found in proving to produce skin rash and irritation in full strength. **Arsenicum album** in very dilute form works for dry and itchy or tender and swollen skin that is worse in winter and at night, with severe itching between midnight and 2 a.m. Restlessness and worsening by the application of warmth are frequent. Flabby people whose hands are clammy and sweaty and who want to eat sweets and eggs may respond to **Calcarea Carbonica**, which also helps infants with cradle cap. **Graphites** improves eczema associated with thick dry skin and a honey like discharge, while chronic eczema with heat and sweatiness, often accompanied by craving for ice and oranges, responds to the nosode **Medorrhinum**, which is made from sterilized pus from gonorrheal discharges. **Mezereum**, made from the very irritating bark of the European ornamental shrub mezereon, helps intense eczema with blistering and oozing followed by crusting. Dry and cracked skin with increased itching at night and in a warm bed is helped by a homeopathic dilution of **Petroleum**, especially eczema of the palms. **Psorinum**, made from the vesicles produced by scabies infection, helps eczema with intense itching and scratching to the point of bleeding, and works for people who are chilly and routinely have dry and itchy skin. **Rhus Toxicodendron** helps very itchy and blistering eczema that is improved by movements and the application of warmth, often with craving for cold milk. A long-used skin remedy is **Sulfur**, which helps people with dry, itchy skin made worse by warmth and bathing, especially people who are hot, restless and thirsty for cold drinks.

Endometriosis represents the

inappropriate presence of tissue normally on the inner surface of the uterus (endometrium) in other places, usually attached to the fallopian tubes and ovaries but sometimes to organs outside of the pelvis such as the bladder. This is a major cause of pelvic and back pain, excessive menstrual bleeding and infertility. **Arnica** may be taken for deep-seated pain and a feeling of soreness and being bruised. **Cimcifuga** is used both herbally and homeopathically for pelvic pain, and the homeopathic preparation works best for shooting or camping menstrual pain. **Colocynthis** is effective for cramping abdominal pain, often improved by abdominal pressure or drawing up the knees in the supine position. Pain radiating from the uterus to the back, often causing back arching but improved by standing up, may be helped by **Dioscorea Villosa**, made from a vine native to the Eastern United States. **Lachesis** is used for primarily left-sided menstrual pain, often with large purple clots and sometimes associated with heat and with jealousy. Cramping pain with gas and bloating improved by heat and worsened by cold or pelvic pressure, may respond to **Magnesia Phosphorica**. **Pulsatilla** is one of the chief menstrual remedies, especially for sensitive and emotional women who crave sweets and want to be comforted. Women with pelvic pain, menstrual problems, pain with intercourse, irritability and craving for sweet, sour or salty foods may be helped by **Sepia.**

Fever can arise from a variety of causes, and needs conventional medical evaluation if persistent or prolonged, but can be reduced and attendant discomforts lessened by several homeopathic remedies. **Aconite** is helpful at the very start of a fever, particularly with sudden onset or recent exposure to cold or wind; its best effect is within hours of the onset of fever, in children who are crying or adults who are restless, and in patients with one red cheek and one pale cheek. **Arsenicum album** is often helpful for fever at night, especially between 12 midnight and 2 a.m., and when fever is accompanied by chills, anxiety or restlessness. **Belladonna** is recommended for sudden and severe fever with a hot body, especially the face, but cold feet, along with dilated pupils, red cheeks and face and throbbing headache, light sensitivity or delirium and hallucinations. People who are thirsty and irritable with fever, and who do not want to move, may respond to **Bryonia**. **Chamomilla** helps fever with teething in infants, as well as fever with irritability and one red and one pale cheek. **Ferrum Phosphoricum** is an effective general fever remedy, especially for those who do not otherwise seem sick, although the face may be red and the body warm.

Fever with chills, muscle aches, fatigue, drowsiness, drooping eyelids and posterior head and neck ache may be helped by **Gelsemium**. **Mercurius** helps when fever is worsened by both cold and warm temperatures, and with fever accompanying sore throat and with coated tongue, bad breath and excessive salivation. **Pulsatilla** is often used for weepy, clingy children with fever who want to be held, and for fever improved by open air. People with very high fever who appear to be very ill may respond to **Pyrogenium,** which is prepared from decomposed and infected meat which has been sterilized and is another example of a nosode, or remedy made directly from diseased tissue. **Sulfur** is used for very acute or very long-lasting fevers, often accompanied by rash and great thirst for cold drinks.

Fibroids, uterine fibromas or leiomyomata uteri are not fibrous tissue but are areas of local growth of connective tissue and smooth muscle within the walls of the uterus. They are very common, affecting 50 per cent or more of women, and are not cancerous and often without symptoms, but can cause excessive uterine bleeding, pelvic pain or pain on intercourse and infertility. Homeopathic options to gunecologic surgery for their removal include **Calcarea Carbonica** for overweight women who are sweaty, easily fatigued, feeling overwhelmed by problems and prone to anxiety, and particularly helps fibroids associated with hemorrhage. **Fraxinus Americanus**, made from the bark of the American ash tree, has similar effects, and **Lachesis** helps pre-menstrual abdominal and pelvic pain, particularly when accompanied by heat or aggravated by warmth or in women who are prone to anger and suspiciousness. Severe menstrual bleeding from fibroids may warrant **Phosphorus**, while intermittent pain with excessive menstrual flow and a desire for sweets and to have others around and to be comforted may suggest the use of **Pulsatilla**. **Sabina** is made from the stems and leaves of *Juniperis Sabina* (savin), a shrub related to the juniper tree, and helps heavy bleeding with lower back and sacral pain from fibroids. Women who feel that the uterus is sagging down and may fall out, and who are irritable and want to be left alone or to eat sweet, sour or salty things, may be helped by **Sepia**. **Sulfur** helps fibroids in women who are easily overheated.

Fibromyalgia is a chronic illness of unknown cause involving chronic musculoskeletal pain, tender areas that can trigger pain, poor and nonrestorative sleep and a host of associated conditions including depression, irritable bowel syndrome, premenstrual syndrome, temporomandibular joint (TMJ) dysfunction, chronic fatigue syndrome, the leaky gut syndrome and abnormal intestinal bacteria, chronic infections and in particular *Candida* overgrowth and food allergies and other autoimmune disorders. Despite its many heterogeneous causes, **Arnica** can help with deep and bruising pain and with muscle tenderness, and **Bryonia** improves pain aggravated by movement, especially in irritable people who do not want to move or be touched. **Calcarea Carbonica** may help people who are flabby, chilly and have clammy hands and feet, and who are anxious and irritable and whose musculoskeletal pain is worse with exertion, cold and damp. **Causticum** is used for stiff and sore limbs after overuse and the feeling that muscles are contracted, as well as pain in cold weather that is improved by the application of warmth. **Cimcifuga** helps sore and bruised muscles, back and neck pain and pain worsened by cold, especially when accompanied by hormonal imbalance and depression. **Ignatia** is recommended for tight muscles, spasms and cramps associated with emotional upset or stress, while **Magnesia phosphoric** may help if muscle tightness or spasms are lessened by applying heat. **Nux vomica** helps fibromyalgia in chilly people who are worse in cold weather and better with the application of warmth, and who have constipation, stomach ache or heartburn as well as irritability and fatigue.

Pain that moves from joint to joint, what used to be called "palindromic rheumatism" may respond to **Pulsatilla**, especially if menstrually-related or associated with depression and tearfulness. Fluctuating pain in restless people that is worse in the morning, improves with activity and then worsens with rest or inactivity may warrant **Rhus Toxicodendron.**

Food allergies and sensitivities are just beginning to be clinically understood, and treatment often requires food elimination and sometimes cumbersome diets. Homeopathic desensitization drops are commercially available and sometimes homeopathic remedies will reduce allergic symptoms, but conventional medical treatment should not be neglected in the event of a severe allergic reaction. **Lycopodium** works for food allergies accompanied by abdominal distention and gas, often worse in the evening and associated with an intense desire for sweets. **Nux vomica** helps irritable people with constipation and headaches as well as other digestive symptoms and chilliness. If food sensitivity results in hives or other allergic manifestations on the skin, this may suggest **Urticaurens**.

Food poisoning is usually caused by bacterial toxins in contaminated food, particularly the *Campylbacter, Salmonella* and *Staphylococcus* species. When severe or prolonged, or when accompanied by symptoms other than cramping pain, nausea and vomiting

or diarrhea, emergency evaluation and treatment may be needed. Lesser symptoms may be ameliorated by **Arsenicum album**, chiefly burning diarrhea, nausea and vomiting, chills, abdominal pain, restless and anxiety. **China** helps exhaustion and weakness after a period of diarrhea or vomiting, and the latter is particularly helped by **Ipecacuanha**, especially when there is a sinking feeling in the stomach and vomiting does not relieve nausea. A particular kind of highly dilute mercury, mercuric chloride or **Mercurius Corrosivus**, is helpful for bloody and burning diarrhea, along with alternate chills and sweating. **Nux vomica** is the iconic homeopathic remedy for nausea and vomiting, and is also useful for loose stools that are painful to pass. **Phosphorus** works for this also, especially with abdominal pain or vomiting that are better with cold drinks or food. **Podophyllum** helps explosive diarrhea or diarrhea with mucus in it, while **Veratrum album** has traditionally been used for rice-water stools accompanied by abdominal cramping and forceful vomiting.

Fungal infections include athlete's foot, nail infections, ringworm of the skin or scalp, thrush (fungal infection of the mouth and gums) and vaginitis. The first three usually involve *Tinea* species and the latter two, *Candida* *albicans.* Antifungal agents are often effective but can be toxic, and eradication of the infection sometimes requires a long course of treatment. **Graphites, Silicea, Sulphur** and **Thuja** (*Thujaorientalis* or wormwood, formerly the chief ingredient in the notorious drink absinthe) are recommended for athlete's foot. *Candida* and other yeast infections may also be helped by **Candida Albicans**, a nosode prepared from highly diluted yeast that stimulates the immune system to fight off the infections.

Gallbladder inflammation

(cholecystitis) and gallstones may affect 20 per cent of more of the population, chiefly after the age of 65, and can result in abdominal pain and digestive symptoms. Alternatives to oral treatment with bile acids, shock-wave lithotripsy or surgical removal of the gallbladder include **Berberis vulgaris** (barberry) for colicky pain radiating from the right side, **Calcarea Carbonica** for people who have the traditional gallstone risk factors of "flabby, fair, fortyish, flatulent and female" and **Chelidonium** (*Chelidonium magus* or greater celandine) for abdominal pain after eating fatty foods. **China** has also been used for the digestive symptoms and pain of gallstones and **Colocynthis** is particularly effective for abdominal pain that makes people double over and apply pressure to

the abdomen, especially with anger or suppressed emotion. When pain is relieved by bending over backward and made worse by bending forward or lying down, **Dioscorea** may be specifically effective. Gallbladder pain and bloating with abdominal distention that is worse in the evening and better with warm drinks or rubbing the abdomen may respond to **Lycopodium**. Right-sided abdominal pain and gas, particularly gallbladder spasms, are helped by **Magnesia phosphoric**, and when symptoms come on after spicy foods, alcohol or stimulants like coffee, particularly with nausea or irritability, **Nux vomica** is called for. Pain after rich or fatty food that improves with fresh air or being consoled and looked after may be helped by **Pulsatilla**.

Gout is caused by the deposition in joints and sometimes in the skin of crystals of uric acid that build up from the breakdown of proteins and to a small extent from intake through food and drink. A genetic deficiency or an overload of uric acid can lead to painful attacks of acute arthritis, particularly of the great toe (podagra), and the condition is also associated with diabetes and insulin resistance. Diet and detoxification are often the mainstays of gout prevention, and the conventional medicine drugs that lower uric acid levels are usually used as a later if not a last resort. **Colchicum**, which is made from members of the crocus family, is a specific remedy for gouty joints. **Arnica** can be used for deep and bruising pain in or around a gouty joint, **Belladonna** for red and inflamed joints that are hot and throbbing and are acutely sensitive to being jarred, **Bryonia** for acute pain in people who are irritable and do not want to move and **Ledum** for knee and foot pain that throbs but is better when ice or cold water are applied. **Pulsatilla** is effective for pain that moves from joint to joint, **Rhododendron** helps gout attacks that flare up before a storm and **Sulphur** has been used for gout with burning pain and itching, dry skin and improvement with cold applications and worsening with heat.

Hair loss is usually a normal phenomenon that is often genetically-determined, but can be a consequence of some diseases like lupus or alopecia areata and can be a complication of cancer chemotherapy. Homeopathic alternatives to hair transplantation and a few conventional drugs such as Rogaine include **Arsenicum album**, which helps fearful and restless people with hair loss when under stress and **Ignatia** when hair loss occurs with emotional trauma, loss or grief. **Lycopodium** may reverse premature hair graying and pattern baldness in men, particularly when a sweet tooth or digestive problems are also present, and **Natrum Muriaticum** helps hair loss associated with depression, sensitivity to the sun and salt craving. Hair loss with grief or sorrow in people who are fatigued or mentally exhausted may be helped by **Phosphorus**, and **Sepia** helps hair loss associated with hormonal factors such as menopause and contraceptive use in women. **Silicea** strengthens brittle hair, often associated with chronic illness, coldness and fatigue.

Headache of any severity generally requires medical or neurological evaluation, but the likelihood of a serious structural cause is low in neurologically normal people. Most recurrent headache is due to migraine, with smaller minorities due to tension or scalp and neck muscle contraction, cluster headache and its relatives and medical or eye disorders. Conventional medical treatments for migraine are quite effective but also quite expensive, and prescription pain medications for chronic headache may cause more problems than they solve. Commercial homeopathic combinations are widely available, and many remedies have been successfully used for head pain. **Belladonna** is effective for right-sided throbbing or bursting headache with flushed face, hot skin and cold feet, as well as improvement when lying down in darkness or quiet. **Bryonia** works for left-sided forehead or eye pain that becomes generalized and is associated with nausea, thirst, irritability and desire to be alone. **Calcarea Phosphoric** works for children with posterior headaches, stomach pain, homesickness and irritability, and **Cimcifuga** for women with menstrual migraines, headaches after menopause or severe neck pain with stiffness. **Gelsemium** helps dull, non-throbbing band-like headache with fatigue and blurred vision, often better after urinating. Headaches with back or neck pain beginning after emotional upset or grief may respond to **Ignatia**, while **Iris** (made from the blue flag or *Iris versicolor*) will be better for right-sided headaches with the features of migraine. **Lachesis** helps similar headaches which predominate or begin on the left, or that cause awakening from sleep and burning, congestion or flushing of the face. **Lycopodium** is used for headaches brought on by not eating, as well as right temple or forehead pain that is worse between 4 and 8 p.m. Tension headaches with band-like distribution and vice-like character are helped by **Magnesia Phosphorica**. **Natrum Muriaticum** is effective for migraine, especially triggered by stress, grief or sun exposure, while headaches after head injury are helped by **Natrum Sulphuricum**, the closely-related sodium sulfate. **Nux vomica** is a classical headache remedy, especially in men and when headaches are accompanied by digestive upset and brought on by too much food or alcohol, especially when irritability, constipation and sensitivity to light and sound are present. Women with menstrual headaches will often respond to **Pulsatilla**, especially if the headaches rapidly change location and are worsened by a hot, stuffy environment or improved by open air. **Sanguinaria** (*Sanguinaria Canadensis* or bloodroot) works for right-sided headache that radiates into the right eye, often relieved by vomiting, and similar headaches involving the left eye and left head are helped by **Spigelia**, made from the genuflecting plant or *Spigelia Anthelmia*, a flowering plant that looks as though it is kneeling.

Hemorrhoids affect up to 75 per cent of the population at some time and about a third of people have them chronically. Constipation, the effects of pregnancy and childbirth and genetic predisposition are the main causes, and conventional medical treatment beyond increased fiber in the diet is mainly symptomatic relief with creams and ointments or surgical removal for severe discomfort or bleeding. **Aesculus**, made from the horse chestnut *Aesculus Hippocastum*, is used for poking or stabbing rectal pain that may extend into the back. Large painful hemorrhoids that resemble a bunch of grapes and are associated with diarrhea may improve with **Aloe**. **Calcarea Fluorica** helps with bleeding, itching, constipation and flatulence associated with hemorrhoids. **Ignatia** is effective for stabling rectal pain and spasms that are associated with emotional upset, while **Nux vomica** is effective for hemorrhoid pain associated with headache, irritability and chronic constipation. **Ratanhia** is prepared from the mint-like South American shrub *Krameria Triandra*, and soothes rectal pain that often feels like sitting on glass. Large hemorrhoids that itch and burn and are associated with anal inflammation and feculent odor, especially at night, may be helped by **Sulphur**.

Hepatitis is inflammation of the liver, usually caused by one of several viruses but sometimes resulting from the effects of drugs or toxic chemicals, and also from the effects of alcohol excess. Antiviral drugs and immunosuppressive treatments will sometimes control but rarely reverse the inflammation, and transplantation is sometimes necessary. Homeopathic remedies are less costly and freer of adverse effects, particularly the specific liver remedy. **Cardus Marianus**, made from several members of the thistle family and effective for inflammation of the left lobe of the liver, which causes abdominal or flank pain that is worse when lying on the left side or with breathing or movement.

Chelidonium is used for right-sided rib and diaphragm pain, radiating to the right shoulder, improved by lying on the left side or by eating and associated with jaundice. Sensitivity to touch or pressure along with marked abdominal enlargement indicate the need for **China**, and **Lycopodium** is used for right upper quadrant pain, bloating and flatulence and irritability and craving for sweets. Jaundice and diarrhea with headache and coated tongue, improved by abdominal pressure, may be helped by **Natrum Sulphuricum**, and hepatitis with constipation, cramping abdominal pain, fatigue, irritability and improvement with heat may respond to **Nux vomica**. **Phosphorus** works for hepatitis due to exposure to solvents and chemicals, and **Sulphur** is effective for severe jaundice and diarrhea.

Herpes infections include cold sores and fever blisters from *Herpes simplex* virus 1 and genital sores and blisters from HSV 2. About 90 per cent of the population has antibody evidence of exposure to one or the other of these, and conventional medical therapy can suppress the external manifestations of the infection but not eliminate it entirely. **Arsenicum album** has long been used for cold sores that burn, especially in restless, anxious and perfectionistic people, while people with very painful mouth sores and irritability and chilliness are more likely to

respond to **Hepar Sulphuricus. Mercurius** is used for cold sores with bleeding gums, coated tongue, heavy salivation, bad breath and burning pain, especially at night, while **Natrum Muriaticum** is used for sores that break out during the day, especially in the sun and under stress; such sores are often near the lips, associated with rhagades or mouth fissures and with depression and salt craving; this is particularly effective for chronic genital herpes, as is **Rhus Toxicodendron** when vesicles break down or ooze readily and patients are worse when cold and damp or feel restless. Burning and itching vesicles that are red or inflamed may respond to **Sulphur.**

Hiatal hernia represents the protrusion of part of the stomach through the diaphragm and into the chest cavity, and is one of the chief causes of reflux of stomach acid into the esophagus and resultant *heartburn.* Numerous antacids and acid-reducing conventional medications are available for this problem, but homeopathic **Arsenicum album** is particularly effective for burning discomfort including heartburn, while **Carbo Vegetabilis** helps indigestion, belching and flatulence. **Lycopodium** works for the same symptoms when they are accompanied by anxiety or lack of confidence and are aggravated by tight clothing and worse in late afternoon or evening. Milk intolerance is sometimes helped by sodium carbonate, diluted to make **Natrum Carbonicum**, and inability to tolerate spicy food or alcohol and the digestion-upsetting effects of stress, overstimulation by light and sound or irritation are helped by **Nux vomica**. **Pulsatilla** is particularly effective for heartburn after eating rich or fatty food, particularly in women and people who are tearful when feeling badly and wish to be comforted. **Phosphorus** helps intense heartburn that is transiently helped by cold drinks but then succeeded by nausea. **Sulphur** is recommended for heartburn, belching and diarrhea.

Hypertension refers to elevated blood pressure from a variety of causes or no evident cause at all. There are a host of conventional medical drugs for control of high blood pressure, but homeopathic options include **Argentum Nitricum** for hypertension and anxiety, sometimes associated with a specific event or performance and exemplified by "stage fright" and often associated with intense warmth and cravings for salt and sweets. The sudden onset of high blood pressure, especially with flushed face, dilated pupils, heat and sensitivity to light may be helped by **Belladonna**. A bursting or explosive headache, flushed face and high blood pressure may benefit from **Glonoinum,** which is made from nitroglycerin, especially in the aftermath of sun exposure or alcohol use. **Lachesis** helps high blood pressure in people who are talkative, jealous, suspicious, intense and very warm and do not want anything touching the neck. People who have high blood pressure when emotionally upset and wish to be alone or who have headaches, palpitations and insomnia may respond to **Natrum Muriaticum**. **Nux vomica** is recommended for hypertension when under stress, often associated with irritability and impatience, coldness, constipation and the desire for coffee or alcohol.

Impotence or *erectile dysfunction*

has affected almost every man at some time, and over 20 million men are estimated to have this problem chronically. Conventional medical treatments are well-known and widely used but are expensive and attended by some cardiovascular concerns. **Agnuscastus** is made from the "chaste berry", *Vitex Agnus Castus*, used by Native American, European and Eastern herbalism for centuries for this problem, and particularly effective for men who were formerly highly active sexually and now may have a cold sensation in the genitals, health anxiety and memory problems. Men with sexual interest, lack of daytime erections but nighttime seminal emissions and frequent tobacco craving may be helped by **Caladium**, made from ornamental plants commonly called elephant's ear, angel wing or heart of Jesus. **Lycopodium** is effective for transient impotence due to worry or low self-confidence, while **Selenium** is helpful for impotence after fever or prolonged illness. Mild-mannered, shy men with repressed emotions or suppressed anger may respond to **Staphysagria**, especially if impotence is related to an embarrassment.

Influenza or flu is an acute viral respiratory infection that is usually benign but can be disabling, and has been catastrophic at times in past epidemics or for patients with compromised immune function or systemic illnesses. There are few conventional medical treatment options, but **Aconite** is effective if taken within hours of the onset of flu symptoms. **Arsenicum album** helps with cold symptoms, diarrhea and vomiting and exhaustion and chilliness, while **Belladonna** is used for sudden onset of flu symptoms with high fever, flushed face, dilated pupils, throbbing headache and hot skin but cold feet. Flu with severe joint pain, irritability and marked aggravation by movement with the desire to remain still is likely to be helped by **Bryonia**. **Eupatorium perfoliatum** or feverwort has long been used for fever in herbal medicine, and in homeopathic form is effective for high fever, muscle aches and thirst, while people with flu who do not seem to be very sick may improve with **Ferrum Phosphoricum**, particularly in taken right away. **Gelsemium** works for flu with muscle aches, chills, headache and drooping eyelids. Flu that is worse when cold or when hot, and with coated tongue, bad breath, increased saliva production and sore throat may respond to **Mercurius**, and flu with prominent digestive symptoms, chilliness and irritability may respond to **Nux vomica**. **Oscillococcinum**, which is made from the hearts and livers of Barbary ducks, is the best-selling homeopathic product and has been shown in controlled studies to alleviate viral illnesses including influenza, if taken at the onset of symptoms. Flu with muscle stiffness that improves with movement but worsens when inactive for a time, or is accompanied by restlessness in bed, may warrant a trial of **Rhus Toxicodendron**. Flu that has been present for a long time may be resolved by **Sulphur**.

Insomnia is a very common complaint, and many of the conventional medical drugs used for its treatment lose their effectiveness after a time and may actually cause worsening of sleep problems, while others can be habit-forming or interfere with alertness. **Aconite** will lessen the acute insomnia that comes with a terrifying event or a sudden emotional or physical shock. People who are fastidious, insecure, anxious or fearful may have trouble sleeping, especially between midnight and 2 a.m., and may fall asleep more easily with **Arsenicum album**. **Cocculus** works for people who have stayed awake for a long time and then cannot fall asleep even though very tired, while **Coffeacruda** helps people who cannot get to sleep because they are over stimulated, typically being awake with thoughts racing at around 3 a.m. **Ignatia** is effective for insomnia due to grief, bereavement or emotional upset, often with uncontrollable crying or sighing during the day, muscle twitching, mood swings and loss of appetite. Insomnia due to overwork and physical or mental exhaustion may be helped by **Kali Phosphoricum**, which works best for people who are anxious and depressed. **Lycopodium** is effective for insomnia attended by fear and low confidence as well as gas, bloating and a desire for sweets. People who cannot sleep after eating or drinking too much, or who sleep restlessly and awaken around 3 a.m. and are then irritable during the day, may be helped by **Nux vomica**. Inability to sleep because of skin or scalp itching or becoming too hot at night has responded to **Sulphur**, while people who have restless legs and muscle jerks at night get relief from zinc (**Zincum Metallicum**).

Irritable bowel syndrome may affect 20 to 30 per cent of the population, both male and female although women are about twice as likely to seek medical treatment for it. It is the most common reason for gastroenterology consultation and involves erratic and irregular rhythmic contraction of the intestines and increased central nervous system sensitivity to pain. There are multiple potential causes and associated conditions, and medical treatment is not always satisfactory. Many homeopathic remedies have been used, including **Argentum Nitricum** for gas, diarrhea and anxiety, often triggered by eating sweets. Diarrhea and burning pain, restless, coldness and nocturnal bowel symptoms may be helped by **Arsenicum album**. **Colocynthis** helps cutting abdominal pain and a feeling of bowel constriction, often helped by bending over and sometimes related to suppressed anger. Abdominal distention and audible bowel gurgling, worse between 4 and 8 p.m. and improved by warmed beverages and accompanied by irritability and low self-esteem as well as craving for sweets may respond to **Lycopodium**. **Magnesia phosphoric** is used for abdominal cramps and muscle spasms that improve when warmth is applied. **Natrum Carbonicum** (sodium bicarbonate) helps indigestion, heartburn and food allergy symptoms, often triggered by dairy products and sweets and in people who wish to be left alone. **Nux vomica** helps abdominal pain and constipation in people with a poor diet or ongoing stress, often worsened by overeating or using stimulants and alcohol. People who are awakened in the morning by diarrhea but have constipation, very smelly gas and rectal irritation, itching and burning may respond to **Sulphur.**

Kidney stones affect up to 10 per cent of American men, and are largely due to hereditary predisposition or to relatively unhealthy diet, and medical treatment consists mostly of pain management, with lithotripsy and surgical removal being used for recurrent cases. Several homeopathic remedies may help to reduce pain without the problems sometimes caused by prescription pain medicines, and others make the formation of stones, which are principally calcium oxalate, less likely. **Belladonna** is effective for sudden excruciating right-sided pain, with fever and flushed face. **Berberis vulgaris** helps more widely distributed pain of shooting or stitching character, while pain that is relieved by bending backward rather than forward may respond to **Dioscorea. Lachesis** is used for left-sided pain and for blood in the urine. Pain in the back or in the abdomen, mostly on the right and worse between 4 and 8 p.m., is an indication to take **Lycopodium**. **Nux vomica** works for kidney colic accompanied by stomach camping, nausea or vomiting, often attended by constipation and irritability.

Lupus refers to a group of disorders in which antibodies are made to the DNA of skin cells (discoid lupus erythrmatosus) or the cells of various internal organs (systemic lupus erythematosus). The disorder is increasing in incidence and predominates in women, particularly African-American, Asian and Hispanic women. Conventional medical treatment involves corticosteroids and immunosuppressive drugs, which are sometimes necessary for severe autoimmune inflammation, but several homeopathic remedies may help to alleviate symptoms. **Arsenicum album** is helpful for burning joint pain improved by warm applications, especially in anxious and restless people. The sudden onset of hot, red, swollen and throbbing joints, worse with motion and sometimes accompanied by fever, may warrant **Belladonna**. Women who have flares of lupus symptoms during menstrual periods, in association with the symptoms of premenstrual syndrome and after menopause may respond to **Sepia**, and symptoms that wander from joint to joint, especially in menstruating or menopausal women, may be helped by **Pulsatilla**. **Rhus Toxicodendron** is effective for joint pain and stiffness improved with motion and worse with activity, especially if cold makes this worse and warmth makes it better. Burning pain improved by the application of cold in someone who gets overheated easily and craves very cold drinks and spicy food may suggest benefit from **Sulphur.**

Menopause is a normal part of the female life cycle but is often treated as a disease by conventional medicine, and the hormone replacement that has been the backbone of such treatment may cause problems and adverse effects. **Belladonna** helps hot flashes and flushing, especially when they begin suddenly and are accompanied by throbbing headache, especially right-sided, restlessness or palpitations. Night sweating, heavy menstrual flow, coldness attended by hot flashes, anxiety, fatigue, a feeling of being overwhelmed, leg cramps and weight gain are associate with response to **Calcarea Carbonica**. Symptoms that are worse when women lie on the left side are helped by **Lachesis**, which also helps women who are talkative, have strong and often negative emotions, experience increased libido, have heart palpitations and cannot tolerate the neck being touched. **Natrum Muriaticum** helps headache and backache with depression, withdrawal from others and tearfulness, sometimes with salt craving and intense thirst as well. **Oöphorinum** is a sarcode, a homeopathic remedy made from healthy tissue, as compared to a nosode made from diseased tissue; oophorinum is prepared from ground ovarian tissue and is a specific remedy for hot flashes after removal of the ovaries. **Pulsatilla** helps menopausal symptoms in tearful women with changeable moods and with aggravation in warm rooms and improvement in fresh air; there is often a strong craving for sweets as well. Craving for sweets and menopausal symptoms are also the hallmarks of benefit from **Sepia**, but this works best for women with prolapsed of the uterus, stress urinary incontinence, irritability, exhaustion and aversion to sexual intercourse as well. Hot flashes and night sweats along with thirst for cold drinks may suggest the use of **Sulphur**.

Motion sickness affects about a third of people who travel, and can be controlled with over-the-counter drugs and if severe by prescription medications that antagonize the serotonin pathways in the brain; the former generally cause sleepiness, and the latter are expensive. Homeopathic combinations for nausea and motion sickness are commercially available. **Borax,** a homeopathic dilution of the sodium borate used in soap, is particularly helpful for nausea with downward motion, as in an airplane, while **Cocculus** helps nausea from forward or rotary motion, as in a car or boat, and for nausea worsened by the smell of food, improved by fresh air and precipitated by sleep deprivation. **Petroleum** helps nausea triggered by rising motions and with a sinking feeling in the stomach, and is particularly helpful for seasickness. Nausea with dizziness, sweating, and faintness triggered by any motion and lessened by cool air is also helped by **Tabacum,** which is prepared from dried tobacco.

Multiple sclerosis is a progressive neurological disease involving inflammation and the formation of scars or plaques in the white matter of the brain and spinal cord. There were very few treatment options for a long time, and conventional drugs may be cumbersome and expensive to use. **Agaricus,** which is made from otherwise poisonous mushrooms and is sometimes called "fly agaric" because it is what makes fly paper sticky, helps with involuntary movements, muscle spasms and impaired coordination as well as abnormal eye movements. Progressive paralysis, confusion, heaviness and sensory loss in the legs and constipation may indicate benefit from **Alumina,** while incoördination and poor balance alone may respond to **Argentum nitricum**. **Arsenicum album** will help paralysis and burning pain, especially in anxious and restless people, while slowly progressive limb weakness, impairment of speech and swallowing, hand and foot numbness and urinary incontinence may respond to **Causticum**. Dizziness, vertigo and loss of visual accommodation along with motor deficit may be helped by **Cocculus. Conium** is used for lower extremity weakness and heaviness with a tendency to drop objects, while **Gelsemium** may be helpful for weakness plus tremor, numbness of the face and tongue, double vision and heavy eyelids. The onset or worsening of multiple sclerosis after grief or emotional trauma, especially with muscle twitching and spasms, may suggest the use of **Ignatia. Natrum Muriaticum** is effective for clumsiness and incoördination with numbness, visible inflammation of the optic nerve (optic neuritis), depression and withdrawal, all of which are made worse by sun exposure. **Nux vomica** helps weakness with muscle spasms and cramps, especially in driven people who may overuse alcohol and coffee or other stimulants. Hand and foot numbness with incontinence and visual loss may be helped by **Phosphorus,** while weakness, heaviness and muscle wasting which predominates in the legs may be improved by **Plumbum**, made from ground lead.

154

Muscle cramps and aches are almost universal and usually benign, but can indicate neurological or medical disorder and should have these evaluations if persistent. There are few options for conventional drug treatment, but **Arnica** is widely used for muscle soreness and **Calcarea Carbonica** may help this in people with cramps and soreness in cold damp climates and are chilly, anxious, easily overwhelmed or fatigued, crave sweets and eggs and have sweaty hands and feet. Stiffness and soreness that is worse in cold dry weather and better with warmth or humidity may respond to **Causticum**. Cramps and soreness in association with hormonal imbalance, menses or depression may be helped by **Cimcifuga**. **Ignatia** helps tight muscles or cramping and soreness triggered by emotional upset and grief. If application of warmth lessens cramps, **Magnesia phosphoric** may be an appropriate remedy. Muscle spasms that are worse with cold and better with warmth and are accompanied by irritability, fatigue and digestive upset suggest **Nux vomica**. If cramps and soreness are improved by activity but increase with rest, are worse in the morning and in cold wet weather and are accompanied by restlessness, **Rhus Toxicodendron** may be helpful.

Obesity is one of the greatest public-health problems and there are few conventional medical drugs to treat it, most of them appetite suppressants that are related to amphetamine and are therefore controlled substances. **Calcarea Carbonica** works best for flabby people who are cold and sweaty, want dairy products and sweets and are easily exhausted or overwhelmed. **Ignatia** lessens comfort eating in sensitive people who are emotionally upset or grieving, and **Pulsatilla** decreases craving for sweets in sad and tearful people who want to be consoled. People with histories of physical or sexual abuse and chronic or repressed anger may eat compulsively, and this can be helped by **Staphysagria**.

Osteoporosis affects about half of American women between 45 and 70 years of age, and reflects the paucity of physical activity and excess of dietary salt and sugar common in modern life, loss of the protective effects of estrogen in women after menopause, increasing incidence of a dysfunctional immune system, the increasing stress of modern life and a significant hereditary component. Conventional medical treatment involves hormone replacement and calcium supplementation as well as newer drugs to facilitate calcium storage in bone, some of them costly. The combination of homeopathic remedies with diet, lifestyle changes and nutritional supplements has been shown to be effective for preventing osteoporosis. The cell salts described above are especially effective for disorders of calcium metabolism: **Calcarea Carbonica** rectifies calcium imbalance, especially in the chilly, flabby, easily fatigued people with symptoms aggravation by cold and damp for whom it generally works, while **Calcarea Phosphoric** can be used to enhance bone building even without other symptoms and works best in people who are discontented and have a desire for travel or change. **Phosphorus** is effective for tall, thin people, often suggestible and social, with a frequent thirst for cold drinks. **Silicea** helps thin people with decreased bone density, especially if nervous, serious, easily exhausted and prone to recurrent infections. **Symphytum** expedites the healing of pathological as well as natural fractures, and can reduce bone pain.

Parasitic infections are among the leading causes of death in developing countries, but are not uncommon in the United States. Many of the conventional drugs used for worm and other infestations must be taken for long periods and may have side effects. **Cina** (*Artemesia Cina* or wormseed) is specifically used for pinworms, accompanied in children by irritability, resistance to being touched, teeth-grinding at night, pallid complexion and increased appetite. **Filix mas** is made from the fern *Dryopteris Filix-mas* and is specific for tapeworms, often associated with swollen lymph nodes, aching nose, dark circles under the eyes and irritability. **Natrum Phosphoricum** (sodium phosphate) works for worms of all kinds, especially when heartburn is present and with a yellow-coated tongue. Intense rectal itching may warrant a trial of **Sabadilla,** rectal itching with bad breath and pain around the navel may be helped by **Spigelia** and **Teucrium,** prepared from the leaves of germander, a member of the mint family, works for worms of all types, attended by rectal itching, irritability and crawling sensations in the nose and rectum.

Parkinson's disease is one of the most common degenerative diseases of the nervous system, and is increasing in incidence as the population grows older. Many conventional therapies are available, but may lose effectiveness with time or produce confusion or excessive involuntary movements instead of the customary rigidity, slowness and tremor. **Argentum nitricum** helps with imbalance, loss of coordination, tremor and deterioration of handwriting (micrographia). **Causticum** works for slowly progressive paralysis, particularly on the right side, and tremor of the hands. Tremor, slurred speech, inability to move the eyes voluntarily and staggering gait are helped by **Gelsemium**, while **Helleborus** is effective for soft and rapid speech as well as mental slowness. **Mercurius** also helps with impaired speech as well as hand tremor, and **Natrum Muriaticum** improves tremor when writing, the tendency to drop objects and decreased expression of emotions. When weakness is slowly progressive and muscle wasting and cramps are present, **Plumbum** may help, while muscle stiffness with little tremor and difficulty starting to move that improves once in motion will respond to **Rhus Toxicodendron.**

Peptic Ulcer Disease was at one time ascribed largely to stress, and conventionally treated with surgery. It is now clear that infection with *Helicobacter pylori* plays a large role in ulcer formation, and courses of antibiotics and medications to reduce acid content are the focus of drug therapy. Homeopathic options include **Arsenicum album** for burning stomach pain that is alleviated by drinking milk, often attended by anxiety and restlessness, **Lycopodium** for pain with gas and bloating that is worse in the afternoon and evening and that is aggravated by wearing tight clothing and **Nux vomica** for symptoms made worse by alcohol, spicy foods and stress, accompanied by constipation and oversensitivity to stimuli. **Pulsatilla** alleviates ulcer pain if related to fatty foods, particularly in those who are sad or tearful when ill, and **Phosphorus** and **Sulphur** both help burning stomach pain, the former when cold drinks lessen the pain but then produce nausea, and the latter when diarrhea is also present.

Poisoning - The best way to deal with *poisoning* is to contact a Poison Control center, and to seek emergent medical attention if symptoms are acute and severe or if the toxic agent is either unknown or known to be a prescription drug, carbon monoxide, insecticide or household chemical. Certain homeopathic remedies, in higher doses such as 30C and taken four times a day, may help with poisoning symptoms from contaminated food, some medications and alcohol excess. **Nux vomica** will help with nausea, vomiting, mental status changes including irritability and gastrointestinal symptoms like constipation. Nausea, vomiting and diarrhea after eating potentially contaminated food may improve with **Arsenicum album.**

Pregnancy is of course not a disease, but is a situation in which many of the conventional medical drugs used for various illnesses and problems are not or may not be safe to use. Pain, especially in the back or sacrum, is frequent and may respond to **Aesculus**, usually when it is worse when sitting and radiates into the right hip. **Arnica** helps with general bruising pain and soreness on moving, while **Bryonia** alleviates pain and stiffness that are worse with movement, aggravated by cold and dry conditions and feel better when the limb is rubbed. **Calcarea Carbonica** helps chronic back pain and weakness in women who are overweight, especially if they feel cold and symptoms are worse in cold and dampness. Back pain and muscle cramps when emotionally upset may be helped by **Ignatia**, and **Magnesia phosphoric** may help with back pain and muscle spasms otherwise, especially if they improve with warmth. **Nux vomica** helps back pain worsened by cold and improved by warmth, especially when chilliness, irritability and constipation are also present. Muscle sprains and strains of ligaments are particularly helped by **Rhus Toxicodendrom**, while pain in the neck and upper back, particularly when worse at night or with limbs that feel weak and lame, may respond to **Ruta**. Other pregnancy-related problems may include swollen bleeding gums, sometimes accompanied by excessive salivation and bad breath, which are helped by **Mercurius**. Bleeding and inflammation are also reduced by **Ferrum Phosphoricum.** Constipation is a

161

frequent complaint, and **Sepia** helps hard and painful stools with a heavy sensation in the abdomen and rectum, often accompanied by irritability, chilliness and a craving for sweets. **Nux vomica** is also effective for constipation attended by urgency and is particularly helpful for pregnant women who feel stressed, work too hard, exercise too little and may eat and drink too much. **Natrum Muriaticum** alleviates constipation associated with depression, sensitivity to light, thirst and craving for salt, and may also help the edema that many women develop during pregnancy. Constipation attended by flatulence and distention of the abdomen, often worse in the late afternoon, is often helped by **Lycopodium**.

Digestive upset including gas and heartburn are frequent, and several homeopathic remedies may relieve these, chiefly **Magnesia phosphoric, Carbo Vegetabilis, Lycopodium** and **Nux vomica**. Stomach pain may be helped by **Arsenicum album**, especially if drinking milk lessens the pain, while difficulty digesting dairy products may be helped by **Natrum Carbonicum**. Stomach upset after fatty food is improved by **Pulsatilla**, especially when mood is often depressed and tearful, and burning in and around the stomach may be alleviated by **Phosphorus** if it is accompanied by nausea or vomiting, or by **Sulphur** if it is accompanied by diarrhea. Hemorrhoids are frequently worse during pregnancy, and **Aesculus** may help them if accompanied by back pain like being poked with a stick, while **Aloe** is effective for large grape-like hemorrhoids and **Calcarea Fluorica** helps hemorrhoids attended by constipation or bleeding. Stabbing or sticking pain and spasms of the rectum may be helped by **Ignatia**, and pain straining at stools due to constipation may respond to **Nux vomica**. Sharp pain after bowel movements may be helped by **Ratanhia**, and nighttime hemorrhoid pain that is associated with a red and irritated anus is improved by **Sulphur.**

Insomnia is common during pregnancy, but prescription sleep medications are generally not recommended. **Coffea Cruda** is effective for overstimulated women who find themselves awake in the middle of the night with racing thoughts, **Ignatia** helps with insomnia due to loss or grief or emotional upset and **Kali Phosphoricum** is effective for insomnia at night due to stress or overwork during the day. Sleep problems related to anxiety, perfectionism, fears and insecurities or to obsessional tendencies may be helped by **Arsenicum album**, and pregnant women who cannot sleep because they are hot or itchy at night may get relief from **Sulphur. Magnesia phosphoric** may help leg restlessness that interferes with sleep, and can relieve leg cramps during the day.

The chief prescription drug used for morning sickness was removed from the market several years ago for fear of class-action lawsuits occasioned by adverse effects on pregnancy. Natural alternatives including homeopathic preparations may be equally effective, including **Ipecacuanha** for constant nausea that is not relieved by vomiting, **Nux vomica** for nausea and vomiting attended by constipation and heartburn, **Colchicum** for nausea triggered by the smell or sight of food and **Tabacum** for nausea brought on by movement.

Pre-eclampsia or toxemia of pregnancy is a disorder of unknown cause that causes hypertension, swelling, protein in the urine and often increased neuromuscular excitability during pregnancy. Its full-blown form can be dangerous to mother and baby and requires obstetrical intervention. Homeopathic **Apis** can help with limb swelling and proteinuria, while water retention and edema, often accompanied by salt craving and heat intolerance, may respond to **Natrum Muriaticum. Sepia** helps pre-eclamptic women who are sad and chilly and who crave chocolate, while **Lachesis** is effective for hypertension, heat and flushing.

Premenstrual syndrome (PMS), sometimes called Late Luteal Phase Dysphoric Disorder, may affect up to 75 per cent of menstruating women. The emotional and physical changes caused by this hormonal disorder were for a long time dismissed as unavoidable if mild and psychologically-based if severe, and the conventional medical treatments of hormone supplementation and antidepressants may be attended by side effects. Homeopathic combination formulas are commercially available, and **Bovista**, made from the spores of puffball mushrooms, is effective for swelling and puffiness as well as awkwardness, clumsiness and dropping objects. **Calcarea Carbonica** helps fatigue, anxiety, overwhelmed feelings, water retention and breast tenderness in association with irregular or prolonged periods. Severe menstrual pain, anger and aggravation of pain by warmth but improvement with motion are hallmarks of likely benefit from **Chamomilla**. **Cimcifuga** is effective for menstrual cramps, shooting pain involving the legs and thighs and headache, neck stiffness or back pain. The emotional concomitants of PMS, such as jealousy, suspiciousness, rage and irritability, and feeling hot with intolerance of anything touching the throat, are particularly helped by **Lachesis.** Irritability and the urge to cross the legs because of the persistent feeling that pelvic and abdominal organs will prolapsed are indications for **Lilium**, which is prepared from *Lilium Tigrinum*, the tiger lily. **Lycopodium** works for PMS with digestive upset, and women who respond are often irritable and bossy but really lack self-confidence, as well as having a large appetite and a sweet tooth. **Natrum Muriaticum** helps menstrual symptoms associated with depression and loneliness, which are aggravated by consolation or sympathy and accompanied by headaches with migrinous features. Impatience, anger and irritability during menses, along with constipation and a desire for alcohol, coffee and foods that are spicy or fatty, suggest benefit from **Nux vomica**. **Pulsatilla** is the most widely used remedy for PMS with emotional symptoms and mood swings, especially with tearfulness and the desire for attention, often attended by a strong desire for chocolate. Similar symptoms plus breast pain and a bearing-down feeling in the uterus but lessened symptoms with exercise are indications for **Sepia.**

Prostate enlargement (hypertrophy) is

present in about half of men over the age of 45, and can be an early sign or prostate cancer that may require urologic evaluation and treatment or the cause of vexing urinary symptoms for which conventional medical treatment is limited. **Apis** is an effective homeopathic option for stinging pain on urination, sometimes accompanied by urinary retention. **Causticum** is recommended for urinary dribbling with coughing or sneezing, and when a pressure sensation is felt between the prostate and the bladder; it also helps restore absent or diminished orgasm. **Chimaphilla** is effective for urinary retention, often accompanied by feelings of sitting on a ball or having a ball lodged in the pelvis. **Clematis**, derived from the otherwise-toxic leaves of the Western or white clematis, alleviates slow urine passage and dribbling, and **Lycopodium** is particularly effective for sexual dysfunction, especially when accompanied by gas, bloating and a desire for sweets. **Pulsatilla** works for bladder pain after urination, particularly in men who easily get too warm and feel better in fresh air. **Sabal Serrulata** (saw palmetto) is used both in homeopathy and herbal medicine for urinary retention and recurrent urinary tract infections. **Selenium** helps both slow urination and dribbling on the one hand and impotence on the other, often with urinary symptoms after urination or walking. Burning on urination, impotence and suppressed emotions or anger are indications for **Staphysagria**, and **Thuja** works particularly for enlarged prostate, urinary frequency and visible forked stream of urine. Prostatism is often associated with painful *prostatitis*, often from infection with fungus, virus or mycoplasma so that antibiotics are ineffective. In addition to the above remedies, **Medorrhinum** may be effective in men who have had gonorrhea or multiple sexual partners, and **Sulphur** is recommended for urethral or prostate burning with back pain, worse after sex or when standing up.

Psoriasis is characterized by plaque-like accumulations of excessive skin cells, sometimes associated with blisters (pustular psoriasis) and also with an arthritis resembling rheumatoid arthritis. Older conventional medical treatments were often applied topically and could be cumbersome, while newer drugs are often expensive and sometimes have significant adverse effects. **Arsenicum album** helps with dry, scaly, itching and burning skin improved by the application of warmth; people who will respond to it are often anxious, precise and fastidious. **Calcarea Carbonica** works for psoriatic plaques that often crack open, particularly in overweight people who are cold but have sweaty hands and feet, and who are often fatigued and anxious. Plaques that ooze fluid and predominate on the scalp, ears, hands and genitals may be helped by **Graphites**, particularly if symptoms are worse at night. People with psoriasis who seem formal and introverted but with closer acquaintance are emotional impulsive, or who have moist or greasy-looking skin, are sensitive to changes in temperature and get skin infections readily, may respond to **Mercurius.** Psoriasis with extremely dry skin, nighttime itching and worse symptoms in the cold and at night may be helped by **Petroleum. Rhus Toxicodendron** works for dry, red skin that is very itchy and people with psoriasis who improve with warmth or hot baths, crave cold milk and feel restless. Skin thickening, breaking out in a circular pattern, dryness, coldness and irritability may suggest benefit from **Sepia**, especially in women with menstrual problems. Psoriasis on the scalp may be improved by **Staphysagria**, and psoriasis with itching, burning and psoriatic arthritis may respond to **Sulphur.**

Another common skin condition is ***Rosacea***, an inflammatory disorder affecting the nose, cheeks, forehead and sometimes chin that causes an initial pink blush and later progressive redness and dilation of blood vessels in the skin. Conventional drug treatment may require taking antibiotics continuously for long periods. **Arsenicum album** can also help dry and flaky skin, especially in cold or restless individuals. Local infections that are tender and drain pus but are improved by warm compresses may also get better with **Hepar Sulfuris.** In females, rosacea often begins at puberty and is aggravated by menses and at menopause, and **Pulsatilla** may be helpful for this. More severe hormone-related symptoms with irritability, fatigue and craving for chocolate, salt and sour foods may respond to **Sepia**. Chronic rosacea or redness worsened by the sun or by hot baths and showers in people who prefer cool climates and want cold drinks may be helped by **Sulphur**.

Shingles is another herpes virus infection, this one caused by *Herpes zoster*, which is the virus that under the name of *Varicella* causes chicken pox. Several antiviral drugs work variably well to suppress the appearance or reappearance of the characteristic vesicles and severe nerve pain of the disorder, and conventional treatment of post-herpetic neuralgia may require the recurrent or long-term use of anticonvulsant or pain-relieving medications. **Arsenicum album** may also help burning pain with itching, worse between midnight and 2 a.m. and better with warm applications, particularly in the anxious or fastidious people who tend to respond to this remedy. When pain has a stinging character and is better with cold and worse with warmth, **Apis** may be helpful. **Iris versicolor** works for right-sided shingles eruptions accompanied by nausea or burning stomach pain. The most severe pain and red irritated skin eruptions may respond to **Mezereum**, and when shingles vesicles are confined to the front or the back of the ribcage, **Ranunculus bulbosus** (buttercup) is effective. **Rhus Toxicodendron** works for an itchy rash with burning pain, improved by warm applications. Burning pain that is better with application of cold and worse with warmth is likely to respond to **Sulphur**. **Variolinum** is a nosode, prepared by dilution of the fluid in a smallpox vesicle, and is used to stimulate the immune system to contain or suppress the shingles eruption.

Sinusitis may be an acute complication of another upper respiratory infection, such as bronchitis, cold or influenza. Chronic sinusitis may be due to obstruction of normal sinus drainage with retention and repeated infection of fluid, environmental or food allergies or the immune response to a chronic fungal infection in the sinus cavity. Conventional treatment consists mainly of surgical drainage or decompression of the sinuses or repeated courses of antibiotics. **Belladonna** may help acute manifestations of fever and throbbing pain, more often on the right side and worsened by bending forward. **Bryonia** may help when head movement is resisted because it is so painful, and **Hepar Sulfuris** may work for a chronically congested and often painful nose, aggravated by drafts. Tenacious yellow or green mucus and pain at the root of the nose may suggest the use of **Kali bichromatum** (bichloride of potassium), and more intense pain in the nose and face with copious saliva, foul-smelling nasal discharge and bad breath may indicate benefit from **Mercurius. Pulsatilla** is effective when thick green or yellow nasal discharge is present, generally better in open air and worse in a warm room. **Silicea** helps recurrent sinusitis with inability to drain, making the sinuses tender but less sensitive when cold is applied.

Sprains of muscles are actually due to damage to a fibrous ligament by undue stretching during physical activity, and cause immediate acute pain with later soreness and swelling. _Strains_ represent damage to muscle fibers from overuse, followed by spasm and pain when an attempt is made to use the muscle again. Conventional treatment involves support, pain relief and the passage of time. **Arnica** is particularly helpful at the onset of pain from either injury, and **Bryonia** lessens pain with movement that limits mobility and causes irritability. Persistent pain and swelling, poor healing of a sprain or strain or susceptibility to recurrent injuries may be helped by **Calcarea Fluorica. Ledum** reduces swelling, particularly in conjunction with the application of ice. Pain that improves with motion but is accompanied by stiffness, and that is alleviated by the application of warmth, may be helped by **Rhus Toxicodendron. Ruta** is also effective for swelling, particularly chronic or after repeated injuries.

Stroke needs to be evaluated emergently and usually treated aggressively in a hospital setting. Some homeopathic remedies may alleviate the severity of neurological deficit or symptoms, and may facilitate later recovery. **Aconite** is helpful for acute agitation, fear and panic in the aftermath of a cerebrovascular event. **Baryta Carbonica** (barium carbonate) may improve mental acuity and behavior problems, and to a lesser extent lessen weakness on either side, while **Causticum** is effective for right-sided neurological deficit accompanied by speech disturbance and sensory loss. **Gelsemium** may help tremor, facial paralysis and drooping eyelids after a stroke, and **Lachesis** has these effects on left-sided symptoms.

Substance use disorder is the most recent name given to alcoholism and drug dependence or addiction. Conventional treatment often focuses on inpatient or outpatient rehabilitation followed by involvement in one or another 12-step support group to achieve and maintain total abstinence from the formerly abused drug, and this is not always practicable or acceptable to the patient. Pharmaceutical treatment for alcoholism, drug withdrawal and cravings may not always be feasible or effective either. **Arsenicum album** helps with these in people who are restlessness, fatigued or anxious, and who may have burning pain lessened by warmth; symptoms are worse between midnight and 2 a.m. **Ignatia** is helps people with emotional labiality, constantly changing mood and symptoms, intense tearfulness but also the strong desire to be left alone, the sensation of a lump in the throat, anxiety and muscle twitches and spasms; they may also harbor long-standing anger and resentment. **Lachesis** works best for people who are angry or violent, or are jealous and paranoid. They are often warm and feel worse in heat, and cannot tolerate anything touching the throat. **Lycopodium** has been particularly used for alcoholism and addiction, especially with irritability and low self-esteem; such patients often feel chilly and are better when warm, crave sweets and have digestive symptoms like gas and bloating. **Nux vomica** is a poisonous excitatory neurotoxin in nature, and may for that reason be particularly useful for excessive nervous excitability in homeopathic dilution; it is particularly effective in withdrawal attended by sensitivity to light and sound, and in people with past or family history of alcoholism. Nausea, constipation, chills and fatigue are other addiction-related symptoms that suggest its use. **Sulphur** has been used for people with alcohol craving and binge drinking, often associated with skin rashes, craving for spicy foods and undue warmth alleviated by cold air and drinks.

Temporomandibular joint dysfunction (TMJ) is an increasingly-recognized cause of face and jaw pain as well as headache, and is often treated conventionally with orthotic devices, orthodontia, dental procedures or jaw surgery, or managed medically with pain medication or anti-inflammatory drugs. **Arnica** can be used for sore and bruising pain in the face or jaw. **Hypericum** is effective for nerve pain with a shooting or radiating character, and **Ignatia** for jaw pain and tight facial muscles in association with situational stress or emotional trauma. **Kali Phosphoricum** also helps with stress and nerve pain, usually with less definite tightness of face and jaw muscles and with less definite shooting pain. **Magnesia phosphoric** is effective for cramps and muscle spasms in the face and jaw. Jaw pain that improves with opening and closing the mouth and then recurs after a period of inactivity, or that is helped by the application of warmth, may respond to **Rhus Toxicodendron**.

Thyroid disease involves overproduction of thyroid hormone (hyperthyroidism) or an under functioning gland (hypothyroidism). Radioactive ablation or surgical removal of the overactive gland is the usual conventional treatment for hyperthyroidism, and hypothyroidism usually requires long-term replacement of thyroid hormone. **Calcarea Carbonica** may enhance thyroid function, which is manifested as coldness, fatigue and difficulty coping and feeling overwhelmed, particularly in flabby people with nighttime sweating. A right-sided goiter with irritability, chilliness, desire for sweets and gas and abdominal distention may be helped by **Lycopodium**. Low thyroid function along with fatigue, coldness, aching, constipation and irritability may be helped by **Nux vomica**. **Pulsatilla** enhances thyroid function in women with menstrual or menopausal symptoms, labiality of emotions and especially tearfulness, sensitivity to warmth and desire for cool air. Similar symptoms plus a craving for sweet, salty or sour food may benefit from **Sepia**. Low thyroid function along with fatigue, coldness, aching, constipation and irritability may be helped by **Nux vomica**.

Vaginitis is one of the most common complaints among women, and can result from

176

the atrophic changes of menopause, overgrowth by yeast such as *Candida Albicans*, sexually-transmitted diseases like *Trichomonas Vaginalis* infection, recurrent antibiotic use that eliminates normal vaginal bacteria and permits fungal overgrowth and suboptimal diet or food sensitivities that also foster bacterial or yeast vaginosis. Conventional medical treatment generally involves hormone supplementation or recurrent courses of antibiotics or antifungal drugs. **Borax** is useful for vaginitis with watery discharge, particularly when it occurs in between menstrual periods. Vaginal burning or itching before or after menses may be helped by **Calcarea Carbonica**, especially in women who fit the physical profile associated with this remedy. **Kali Bichromatum** may be effective if thick yellow discharge is present and causes irritation of the external genitalia. The most-often prescribed remedy for vaginitis is **Kreosotum** (creosote, distilled from the tar of the beechwood tree), which works when burning and putrid discharge is associated with itching and is worse during pregnancy or before menses. A discharge resembling egg white with vaginal dryness, sensitivity to the sun and a reserved demeanor are the hallmarks of benefit from **Natrum Muriaticum**. **Pulsatilla** works when discharge is creamier of thicker, and when symptoms are variable throughout the day; a thicker still discharge which is yellow and very odorous, and is accompanied by a bearing-down feeling in the pelvis and by irritability and fatigue, may respond to **Sepia**. When there is itching and burning, and symptoms are worse after bathing and when warm, **Sulphur** may be more effective.

Warts are mounds of overgrown skin on the feet, hands, knees, elbows, genitals and anus that are caused by local infection by many different kinds of virus. They are unsightly and occasionally painful, especially on the feet, but there is little conventional therapy except topical application of acid or freezing and removing them. **Antimonium Crudum** (antimony sulfide) helps with fingertip, nail bed and foot (plantar) warts that are flat and hard. Large warts that bleed and are soft and fleshy, often on arms, face and hands, may respond to **Causticum**, while similar warts on the hand are helped by **Dulcamara**. **Acidumnitricum** (nitric acid) can clear painful cauliflower-shaped warts that sometimes bleed from the anus, genitalia and mouth. Recurrent crops of warts, particularly those that recur after they are surgically excised, frozen or burned off, may respond to **Thuja**.

FURTHER READING

Balch JF, Stengler M (2010). *Prescription for Natural Cures, ed. 2.*Hoboken NJ: JohnWiley& Sons.

Brandl A. (2003). *Homeopathy Pocket.* Hermosa Beach CA: BörmBruckmeier Publishing.

Hahnemann S. (2014). *Organon of Medicine.*Seattle: Amazon Digital Services.

Lockie A, Owen D (2006). *Encyclopedia of Homeopathy, ed. 2.*London: Dorling Kindersley Publishers.

McCabe V (2000). *Practical Homeopathy.* New York: St. Martin's-Griffin.

Sankaran R (2011). *Homeopathy for Today's World.* Rochester VT: Healing Arts Press.

Stengler, M. (2010). *The Natural Physician's Healing Therapies.* New York: Prentice-Hall Press.

Vithoulkas, G. (2014). *The Basic Principles of Homeopathy.*Alonissos: International Academy of Classical Homeopathy.

CPSIA information can be obtained
at www.ICGtesting.com
Printed in the USA
LVOW01s1918180516

488860LV00029B/619/P